Tobacco Cessation and Substance Abuse Treatment in Women's Healthcare

Byron C. Calhoun • Tammi Lewis
Editors

Tobacco Cessation and Substance Abuse Treatment in Women's Healthcare

A Clinical Guide

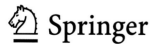 Springer

Editors

Byron C. Calhoun
Department of Obstetrics
  and Gynecology
West Virginia University-
  Charleston
Charleston, WV, USA

Tammi Lewis
Family Resource Center
Women and Children's Division
Charleston Area Medical
  Center
Charleston, WV, USA

ISBN 978-3-319-26708-1   ISBN 978-3-319-26710-4   (eBook)
DOI 10.1007/978-3-319-26710-4

Library of Congress Control Number: 2016933484

Springer Cham Heidelberg New York Dordrecht London

Printed on acid-free paper

Springer International Publishing AG Switzerland is part of Springer Science+Business Media (www.springer.com)

Contents

Contributors

Denise Burgess, RN, BSN, MA, LPC, NBCC Charleston Area Medical Center, Charleston, WV, USA

Byron C. Calhoun, MD, FACOG, FACS, FASAM, MBA Department of Obstetrics and Gynecology, West Virginia University-Charleston, Charleston, WV, USA

Paul Dietz, MD, FACOG Department of Obstetrics and Gynecology, Charleston Area Women's Medicine Center, Medical Center, Charleston, WV, USA

Tammi Lewis, LPC, AADC, SAP Family Resource Center, Women's and Children's Division, Charleston Area Medical Center, Charleston, WV, USA

Chapter 1
Introduction: Abuse of Tobacco and Substances

Byron C. Calhoun

Introduction and Background

The substance abuse rates in the United States have been estimated to be between 2.8 and 19 % [1–3]. The most recent data available (2013 data) reported by the Substance Abuse and Mental Health Services Administration (SAMHSA) in 2015 found a 2.6 % rate of illicit drug use in the United States in 2013 [4]. However, most concerning are the much higher rates of substance use in the reproductive age cohorts. The rates at 12–17 years of age were 3.5 %; the 18–25 years of age an astonishing 7.4 %; and the 26–44 years of age 3.1 %. This data demonstrates the significant public health issue substance abuse and illicit drug use in women's reproductive health particularly in obstetrical care. SAMHSA depends heavily on the use of survey data, self-reporting, and reporting from healthcare entities. The data are not generally linked to actual substance testing or necessarily verified with biologic samples.

B.C. Calhoun, MD, FACOG, FACS, FASAM, MBA (✉)
Department of Obstetrics and Gynecology, West Virginia University-Charleston, Charleston, WV, USA
e-mail: Byron.calhoun@camc.org

© Springer International Publishing Switzerland 2016   1
B.C. Calhoun, T. Lewis (eds.), *Tobacco Cessation and Substance Abuse Treatment in Women's Healthcare*,
DOI 10.1007/978-3-319-26710-4_1

Reported rates vary based upon the population screened and the method of screening used. The lowest number reported in the study by Ebrahim and Gfroerer utilized a population survey of the entire United States [1] while the highest rates reported (19 %) by Azadi and Dildy utilized urine toxicology testing [3]. Chasnoff et al. 2005 developed a screening tool that estimated that 15 % of the population studied continued to use substances of abuse after becoming aware of the pregnancy [2]. The American Congress of Obstetricians and Gynecologists further affirms the validity and necessity of substance use and alcohol abuse screening in women's healthcare:

> Routine screening for substance use disorder should be applied equally to all people, regardless of age, sex, race, ethnicity, or socioeconomic status. Routine screening for substance use disorder can be accomplished by way of validated questionnaires or conversations with patients. Routine laboratory testing of biologic samples is not required [5].

Other screening recommendations in clinical practice that have proved useful include the use of the "4P's" [6]. This screening consists of asking specific questions about Parents (did any of the parents have a drug or alcohol problem); Partner (does their partner have a problem with alcohol or drug use); Past (have you ever had trouble in life because of alcohol or other drugs, including prescription medications); and Present (in the past month have you drunk any alcohol while pregnant or used other drugs) [6]?

Adolescents present a particularly vulnerable population and may need more detailed screening questions about alcohol and drug use with regard to driving, self-esteem, relaxation, interpersonal relations including family, and any type of trouble (school or legal). Adolescents also present issues in confidentiality that must be dealt with in the context of substance abuse. Consultation with various state guidelines and legislation is recommended.

Recent work published by Montgomery et al. 2006 compared the performance of meconium samples versus the testing of umbilical cord tissue [7]. This study showed concordance of the testing methods that correlated at or above 90 % for all substances analyzed in both cord blood and meconium. Follow-up work included a study in which umbilical cord samples were collected and tested if high risk criteria for substance abuse were identified. Out of this cohort, 157 of 498 (32 %) cords tested positive for substances of abuse [8]. Stitely et al. 2010 found similar results in their study of a cohort of blinded umbilical cord blood samples in eight regional hospitals in West Virginia in 2009 with 146/759 (19.2 %) of umbilical cord samples collected at delivery that were positive for either illicit substances or alcohol [9]. In this study, no patient screened positive by risk criteria or admitted to use of any illicit substances or alcohol.

Data from our own state of West Virginia found the number of newborns treated for neonatal abstinence syndrome (NAS) has increased dramatically in our state. In data collected from the Cabell Huntington Hospital in Huntington, WV, the number of neonates treated for NAS increased from 25 in 2003 to 70 in 2007 [10]. Further, the cost difference in the care of an otherwise healthy neonate with NAS compared to a normal full-term healthy neonate was estimated to be $3934 in the Cabell Huntington cohort in 2007 dollars. Because of the added costs associated with the increased risk of prematurity, the average cost of hospitalization in all infants with NAS was $36,000 compared to $2000 for a normal neonate [9]. These hospital costs do not include the substantial increased need for resources to deal with the morbidity of prematurity with regard to additional therapies, medical costs, and burden on families due to prematurity and NAS.

Recent work by Hensel et al. 2012 found with universal urine screening for illicit substances in an obstetric and gynecologic residency clinic in West Virginia that 32 % of pregnant patients were positive for illicit substances including 11 % positive for multiple substances [11]. No patients in the study admitted to, or self-identified as, using illicit drug or ingesting alcohol.

The substance abuse literature previously described the avoidance of detoxification during the second and third trimesters of pregnancy due to concerns about harms to the fetus [12, 13]. These fears included the effects of acute opiate withdrawal on the fetus with possible increased risk of early pregnancy losses or fetal demise in later trimesters [12, 13]. Recent literature, however, does not substantiate these claims [14–16]. Careful detoxification of patients does not appear to increase the risk for early first trimester losses or stillbirths in the later trimesters [14–16]. Luty et al. 2003 studied 101 opiate-dependent women who underwent a gradual, controlled, and supervised 21-day opiate withdrawal with no adverse effects found [16]. Stewart et al. 2013 utilized a slow methadone taper for pregnant inpatients. They found that in 53/96 (56 %) of patients could successfully be detoxified [17]. Further, the hospital stays for patients with inpatient detoxification lasted 10 days longer than those who did not detoxify (25 versus 15 days). They also found that maternal demographics and drug histories did not influence successful detoxification. Their findings suggested that opiate detoxification ought to be offered to all pregnant women willing to undergo detoxification [17].

Finally, Hensel et al. 2015 cared for 92 urine substance screen-positive pregnant patients and achieved abstinence in 39/92 (42 %) patients at delivery with outpatient management with therapeutic substitution with decreasing dosages of oral opiates while including contingency addictions care [18]. They found collaborative and intense group therapy with a certified addictions counselor with the weekly group therapy was a mainstay of successful achievement of abstinence.

In contrast to abstinence in pregnancy, opioid dependence, including methadone maintenance, has been linked to fetal death, growth restriction, preterm birth, meconium aspiration, and NAS [12, 19]. NAS may be present in 60–90 % of neonates exposed in utero with up to 70 % of affected neonates with central nervous system irritability that may progress to seizures [20]. Up to 50 % of neonates may experience respiratory issues, feeding problems, and failure to thrive [21]. These issues are present as well in those infants whose mothers' are on methadone maintenance [22]. However, with methadone, the onset of NAS may be delayed for several weeks [22]. Further, the withdrawal symptoms and signs may mimic other common neonatal maladies: upper respiratory infection, diarrheal diseases, and even colic. This confusion often leads to misdiagnosis and morbidity. Therefore, some authors recommend 5–8 days of maternal hospitalization while their neonates' undergo observation for NAS [23]. However, most insurance plans will not reimburse for the accompanying prolonged uncomplicated maternal stay.

The incidence of opioid relapse in pregnant opioid-abusing women is very high with 41–96 % relapsing [24]. This mirrors the relapse rate of the general population at 1 month of 65–80 % [24, 25]. Over 90 % of patients will relapse at 6 months after medication-assisted withdrawal [26]. Relapse constitutes the most difficult issue to be dealt with postpartum. Improved methods for maintenance of sobriety are sorely needed in the postpartum period and beyond. In spite of the hope of decreased incidence of NAS, Buprenorphine (Subutex™) appears to have no difference in outcomes with regard to treatment of opiate-addicted women. The same NAS and neonatal affects are present [27].

Anomalies associated with opioids appear to be related to first trimester use of codeine and an increased risk of congenital heart defects [28–31]. According to the literature, exposure to oxycodone, propoxyphene, or meperidine have not been linked to increased risk of congenital anomalies [32, 33]. There is a report from a single retrospective study that found an increased risk of birth defects with prescription opioids in women who took these medications in the month before or during the first trimester of pregnancy [34].

Use of heroin in pregnancy has been associated with an increased risk of fetal growth restriction, abruption placentae, fetal death, preterm labor and meconium in utero [35]. It is speculated that these issues arise from the repeated exposure of the fetus to opioid withdrawal and the effects of withdrawal on the placenta. Further, all the risk taking activities the patients engage in such as prostitution, theft, violence, and intimate partner violence accentuate the medical effects of addiction.

According to SAMHSA 2015 (using 2013 data as last completed year of analysis), over 6.9 million people age 12 years or older had illicit drug dependence or abuse [36]. Further, SAMHSA reports the dismal statistic that only 13.4 % (about some 917,000 treated/6.9 million people with a problem) received treatment. Most startling as well was that 8 out of 10 people with illicit drug dependence or abuse did not perceive a need for treatment for their illicit drug use. Considerable disconnect exists between people's perceptions of illicit drug use with addiction and the reality of addiction their lives. It is not clear from the SAMHSA data that treatment is not always available with a lack of services for addictions and mental health or that the individuals have never been questioned or confronted regarding their illicit substance abuse or addiction.

Treatment for alcohol dependence or abuse, according to the SAMHSA 2013 data, appears no better. SAMHSA reports some 17.3 million people greater than age 12 years have been found to have alcohol dependence or abuse [37]. Of that 17.3 million, only 1.1 million (6.3 %) received treatment. Nine out of ten individuals with alcohol dependence or abuse did not perceive a need for treatment for their alcohol use. There was no difference in treatment rates by health insurance status, socioeconomic status, or rural versus urban areas. Once again, perceptions by individuals is sorely lacking regarding the harmful effects of their alcohol dependence or abuse. Also, it is not possible from the SAMHSA data to determine if treatment is not available due to a lack of services for addictions and mental health, or, that the individuals have never been questioned or confronted regarding their illicit substance abuse or addiction.

Tobacco

Tobacco abuse continues to be a major problem among adolescents. SAMHSA 2015 (using 2013 data as last completed year of analysis), reported that 5.6 % of adolescents aged

12–17 (approximately 1.4 million adolescents) admitted to using cigarettes within a month of the 2013 survey [38]. Cigarette usage was also higher in metropolitan areas (8.4 %) compared to rural areas (5.1 %). SAMHSA further reported that the number of US adolescents using cigarettes had dropped from 9.0 to 5.6 % from 2009 to 2013. There were significant drops in usage reported in Whites, Blacks, and Hispanics.

West Virginia leads the nation in the percentage of women who smoke while pregnant (35.7 %) [39]. From 2000 to 2005, while most of the country experienced declines in smoking rates among pregnant women, West Virginia experienced an increase in smoking rates in all stages of reproduction. Smoking rates increased (36.2–45.8 %) prior to pregnancy, (29.4–35.7 %) during pregnancy and (1.6–39.3 %) postpartum [39]. Findings from the West Virginia Bureau for Public Health, Health Statistics Center indicated that during 2005, pregnant women in West Virginia who smoked were 63.2 % more likely than non smoking pregnant women to have their child die during his/her first year of life. In addition, they were 97.4 % more likely to give birth to a low birth weight baby and 282 % more likely to have a child die from Sudden Infant Death Syndrome within his/her first year when compared to those who did not smoke.

Research studies have well established that tobacco dependence during pregnancy increases the risk of poor fetal outcomes. Tobacco use during pregnancy is known to be related to small for gestational age infants (SGA) intrauterine growth retardation (IUGR), low birth weight [40–43], preterm birth [44, 45], and intrauterine death [46]. One study estimated that 5 % of infant deaths in the United States were attributable to maternal smoking while pregnant [47]. Smoking further affects the fetus and includes an increased risk for cryptorchism in males [48], orofacial clefts [49], decreased white cell precursors [50], and increased risk for asthma and bronchopulmonary hyperreactivity [51, 52]. Perinatal morbidities include an increased risk for placental abruption [53] and stillbirth [53–55]. Mental disorders are also increased among women with nicotine dependence [56]. Recently findings about prenatal exposure to tobacco include an association of reduced brain growth in fetuses [57]; significant increase in attention-deficit/hyperactivity (ADHD), oppositional defiant disorder (ODD) and conduct disorder (CD); [58, 59] and risk of poor school performance during adolescence [60].

Multiple perinatal outcome variables have been examined and various conclusions have been drawn regarding the gestational age by which tobacco use should stop to ameliorate its deleterious effects [61]. Researchers examining the effects of smoking cessation during pregnancy concluded that pregnant women who quit during their first trimester had reductions in the proportion of preterm deliveries and low birth weight infants [62]. Another study concluded that maternal third-trimester cigarette use is a strong and independent predictor of birth weight percentile [63]. In examining growth retardation with tobacco exposure, Horta et al. noted that there is a direct dose-response association [64]. It was concluded in another study that if patients stop smoking before 20 weeks that the effects of tobacco may be ameliorated and the fetus will experience normal growth [61]. Further, patients with a previous history of tobacco use with a previous child with intrauterine growth restriction may have normal fetal growth and normal birth weight for their current tobacco free pregnancy [42]. These findings support continued attempts to influence patients to stop smoking even into the mid-trimesters of gestation.

Alcohol

Staff of Charleston Area Medical Center (CAMC), West Virginia's only free-standing Women and Children's Hospital knew they were providing care to around 130 babies born annually with positive substance screens (4 % deliveries) based on risk factor screening at the time of presentation and delivery. However, the actual numbers were much more alarming. We obtained new information for our hospital from Stitely et al. 2010 study of cord bloods that indicated a much higher abuse rate [9]. A cross-sectional hospital study was initiated in eight West Virginia hospitals in 2009 to examine the prevalence of substance use in pregnant patients at delivery and CAMC participated [9]. Segments of umbilical cords were collected anonymously from 759 deliveries (regardless of risk factors) at the eight regional hospitals during the month of August 2009. A reference laboratory screened all cord segments for the presence of substances using commercially available enzyme linked immunoabsorbent (ELISA) kits, with confirmatory testing by gas chromatography/mass spectrometry used for detection of 6 of the illicit drugs. Buprenorphine was tested using liquid chromatography/mass spectrometry (LCMSMS). Phosphatidylethanol (a metabolite of ethanol) testing was based on high pressure liquid chromatography/mass spectrometry (HPLCMS). CAMC's overall positive screening rate was 16 % for non-prescribed and illicit drugs and 8 % for alcohol out of the total of 133 patients screened. These findings were four times higher than our rate of 4 % positive tests when we screened patients based on risk factors alone. In addition, results from the study indicated that multiple drug use was common [9].

Recent screening for alcohol now includes the use of phosphatidylethanol (PEth). PEth is a group of glycerophospholipid homologs formed extrahepatically, in the red blood cell membranes, by the action of phospholipase in the presence of ethanol. PEth groups contain a common nonpolar phosphoethanol head group onto which tow saturated or unsaturated fatty acids, typically with a chain length of 16, 18, or 20 carbons are attached. Several different molecular types of PEth have been identified in blood collected from alcoholic subjects [65–67]. The most abundant subtypes are those containing a saturated fatty acid with a chain length of 16 carbons (PEth 16:0 species) and the 18 carbons and one double bound (PEth 18:1 species) [65, 66]. Kwak et al. 2012, previously reported in a small group of 13 pregnant patients with self-reported alcohol use, the usefulness of the PEth 16:0 and

PEth 18:1 as a reliable biomarker for alcohol ingestion [68]. The most recent study by Kwak et al. 2014 found in their study of 305 patients (117 self-reported users of alcohol/88 abstainers) that there is quantifiable PEth blood concentration after self-reported abstinence period of 3–4 weeks, and a dose-response increment of PEth blood concentrations in relation to alcohol consumption [69]. These findings are consistent with the findings of a half-life of total PEth blood concentration of approximately 4 days in chronic alcoholics while the half-life in healthy subjects varies from approximately 4.5–12 days. Therefore, PEth may be present up to 3–4 weeks after last alcohol ingestion and the correlation may be imprecise regarding last ingestion due to the varying half-life and kinetics in specific patients based on alcohol usage and clearance [70, 71]. Thus, PEth provides a means of screening for alcohol consumption in pregnant patients but should be used cautiously since it may be misleading if patients have only recently stopped using alcohol (within the last 3–4 weeks) upon ascertainment of pregnancy. Repeated samples during pregnancy may be necessary to validate abstinence from alcohol use. Optimal screening for alcohol with PEth in pregnancy and alcohol screening in general in pregnancy have not yet been established.

Amphetamines

Based on findings in humans and the confirmation of prenatal exposures in animals, amphetamines and methamphetamines increase the risk of an adverse outcome when abused during pregnancy. Clefting, cardiac anomalies, brain malformations, renal anomalies, gastroshisis, and fetal growth reduction deficits that have been seen in infants exposed to amphetamines during pregnancy [72–78]. These findings have all been reproduced in animal studies involving prenatal exposures to amphetamines [72]. The differential effects of amphetamines between different genetic strains of mice and between various species demonstrate that pharmacokinetics and the genetic disposition of the mother and developing embryo can have an enormous influence on enhancing or reducing these potential risks [72]. The effects of prenatal exposure to amphetamines in producing altered behavior in humans appear less compelling when one considers other confounding variables of human environment, genetics, and polydrug abuse. In view of the animal data concerning altered behavior and learning tasks in comparison with learning deficits observed in humans, the influence of the confounding variables in humans may serve to increase the sensitivity of the developing embryo/fetus to prenatal exposure to amphetamines. These factors and others may predispose the developing fetus to the damaging effects of amphetamines by actually lowering the threshold of susceptibility at the sites where damage occurs. Knowledge of the effects of prenatal exposure of the fetus and the mother to designer amphetamines is lacking.

Treatment of amphetamine abuse with fluoxetine and imipramine may be useful but is not a panacea for treatment. A recent review by the *Cochrane Collaboration* in 2001 (reissued in 2009) noted that medications are of limited use in treatment of amphetamine abuse [79]. They note that there are very limited trials at this time to be able to suggest the best way to treat amphetamine abuse. Therefore, amphetamine use and abuse proves to be a difficult addiction to treat medically.

Benzodiazepines

Late third-trimester use and exposure during labor and delivery of benzodiazepines appears to be associated with greater risks to the fetus/neonate than earlier exposure in the first and second trimesters. Infants exposed in the third trimester, but by no means all infants, exhibit either the floppy infant syndrome, or marked neonatal withdrawal symptoms. Symptoms vary from mild sedation, hypotonia, and reluctance to suck, to apneic spells, cyanosis, and impaired metabolic responses to cold stress.

These symptoms have been reported to persist for periods from hours to months after birth. This correlates well with the pharmacokinetic and placental transfer of the benzodiazepines and their disposition in the neonate. However, there has been no significant increase in the incidence of neonatal jaundice and kernicterus in-term infants related to benzodiazepine use. The prolonged use of benzodiazepines throughout pregnancy has raised concerns that there may be altered transmitter synthesis and function, leading to neurobehavioral problems in the children. However, it is important to consider poor environmental and social factors when assessing the prenatal influence of the benzodiazepines on the postnatal health and development of the child. There is evidence that clonazepam, clorazepate, diazepam, lorazepam, midazolam, nitrazepam, and oxazepam are excreted into breast milk. The published data indicate that the levels detected in breast milk are low; therefore, the nursing infant is unlikely to ingest significant amounts of the drug in this way. However, problems may arise if the infant is premature or has been exposed to high concentrations of drug either during pregnancy or at delivery.

Benzodiazepine dependence and detoxification must be done gradually to reduce symptoms. Rapid detoxification has been linked to withdrawal seizures. Little has been written about benzodiazepine detoxification in pregnancy.

Marijuana

Animal research suggests that the brain's endocannabinoid system plays a significant role in the control of fetal brain maturation, particularly in the development of emotional responses. Therefore, THC exposure very early in life may negatively affect brain development. Research in rats suggests that exposure to even low concentrations of THC late in pregnancy may cause significant and long-lasting consequences for both the developing fetal brain and behavior of offspring [80]. Human studies have shown that babies born to women who routinely used marijuana during their pregnancies may respond differently to visual stimuli, tremble more, and have a high-pitched cry, consistent with NAS [81, 82]. Children prenatally exposed to marijuana are more likely to show issues in problem-solving skills, memory, and the ability to remain attentive [83, 84]. Further research is needed, however, to separate marijuana's deleterious effects from environmental factors, including maternal nutrition, exposure to nurturing/neglect, socioeconomic status, and use of other illicit substances by pregnant patients [85].

Cocaine

Similar to amphetamines, cocaine has been linked to clefting, cardiac anomalies, limb defects, brain malformations, renal abnormalities, gastroschisis, and fetal growth reduction have been seen in infants exposed to cocaine during pregnancy [72–78]. The differential effects of cocaine between genetic strains of mice and between species demonstrate that pharmacokinetics and the genetic disposition of the mother and developing embryo can have an enormous influence on enhancing or reducing these potential risks [86].

With regard to the long-term neurodevelopmental effects that maternal cocaine use may have on the fetus, a recent systematic review concluded that among children aged 6 years or younger, there is no convincing evidence that prenatal cocaine exposure has effects significantly different from those attributed to other prenatal exposures, including maternal tobacco and alcohol use [87]. However, this remains an area in need of more research with well-designed studies. Subtle developmental delay may be extremely difficult to identify and behavioral issues may not manifest until later in childhood.

Several behavioral treatments for cocaine addiction have proven to be effective in both inpatient and outpatient settings. Indeed, behavioral therapies are often the only available and effective treatments for substance abuse, including stimulant addictions. However, the integration of behavioral and medication therapies may ultimately prove to be the most effective approach. One form of behavioral therapy that is showing positive results in cocaine-addicted populations is contingency management, or motivational incentives (MI). MI may be particularly useful for helping patients achieve initial abstinence from cocaine and for helping patients stay in treatment. These programs use a voucher or prize-based system that rewards patients who abstain from cocaine and other drug use as an incentive to sobriety. On the basis of drug-free urine tests, the patients earn points, or chips, which may be exchanged for items that encourage healthy drug-free living, such as a gym membership, movie tickets, or dinner at a local restaurant. Further, our own program at CAMC used weekly gifts for the patients' pregnancy, while presenting car seats and strollers at the completion of the program. This approach has recently been shown to be practical and effective in community treatment programs.

Cognitive-behavioral therapy (CBT) is an effective approach for preventing relapse. CBT is focused on helping cocaine-addicted individuals abstain — and remain abstinent — from cocaine and other substances. The underlying assumption is that educational processes play an important role in the development and continuation of cocaine abuse and addiction. These same learning processes can be harnessed to help individuals reduce drug use and successfully prevent relapse. This approach attempts to help patients recognize, avoid, and cope; that is, they recognize the situations and triggers in which they are most likely to use cocaine, avoid those situations and triggers when appropriate, and cope more effectively with a range of problems and problematic behaviors associated with drug abuse. This therapy is also useful because of its compatibility with a whole range of other treatments patients may receive.

Therapeutic communities (TCs), or residential programs, offer another alternative to persons in need of treatment for cocaine addiction. TCs usually require a 6- or 12-month stay and use the program's entire "community" of other substance abusers as active components of treatment. They can include onsite vocational rehabilitation and other supportive services and focus on successful re-integration of the individual into society.

Community-based recovery groups—such as Cocaine Anonymous—that use a 12-step program can also be helpful to people trying to sustain abstinence from drugs. Participants may benefit from the supportive fellowship and from sharing with those experiencing common problems and issues.

It is important that patients receive services that match all of their treatment needs. For example, if a patient is unemployed, it may be helpful to provide vocational rehabilitation or career counseling along with addiction treatment. If a patient has marital problems, it may be important to offer couples counseling.

Finally, there are no proven medications to treat cocaine addiction.

Comorbidities

Comorbidities with multiple psychiatric issues in the patients with substance abuse issues must be considered. The 2011 USA National Survey on Drug Use and Health found that 17.5 % of adults with a mental illness had a co-occurring substance use disorder; involving some 7.98 million people [88]. A significant number of patients with substance dependence have affective disorders including: depression, mania, schizoaffective disorders, schizophrenia, borderline personality, and bipolar disorders. A study by Kessler et al. 1994 in the United States, attempting to assess the prevalence of dual diagnosis with substance abuse and mental illness, found that 47 % of patients with schizophrenia had a substance misuse disorder at some time in their life [89], and Regier et al. 1990 found the chances of developing a substance abuse disorder was significantly higher among patients suffering from a psychotic illness than in those without a psychotic illness [90]. Another study looked at the extent of substance abuse in a group of

187 chronically mentally ill patients living in a community setting. According to the clinician's evaluations, about 33 % of the samples used alcohol, street drugs, or both, during the 6 months before evaluation [91].

Therefore, many authors recently note that detoxification must be linked with a combination of behavioral therapy with contingency management therapy to deal with the significant mental health issues associated with substance abuse [23, 92, 93].

Conclusions

Substance abuse in pregnancy presents a significant cost in both maternal, fetal, and neonatal morbidities and mortalities. Subsequent chapters will focus on the physiology of nicotine, alcohol, opiates, and other receptors as well as women's specific issues in addictions, health effects, pregnancy effects, tobacco cessation, addictions counseling, and therapeutic substitution with pragmatic strategies for care.

References

1. Ebrahim SH, Gfroerer J. Pregnancy-related substance use in the United States during 1996-1998. Obstet Gynecol. 2003;101(2): 374–9.
2. Chasnoff IJ, McGourty RF, Bailey GW, Hutchins E, Lightfoot SO, Pawson LL, Fahey C, May B, Brodie P, McCulley L, Campbell J. The 4P's Plus screen for substance use in pregnancy: clinical application and outcomes. J Perinatol. 2005;25(6): 368–74.
3. Azadi A, Dildy III GA. Universal screening for substance abuse at the time of parturition. Am J Obstet Gynecol. 2008;198(5): e30–2. Epub 2008 Feb 14.
4. Substance Abuse and Mental Health Services Administration. Behavioral health barometer: United States, 2014. HHS publication no. SMA-15-4895. Rockville: Substance Abuse and Mental Health Services Administration; 2015. p. 14.

5. American College of Obstetricians and Gynecologists Committee Opinion Number 633: Alcohol abuse and other substance use disorders: ethical issues in obstetric and gynecologic patients; June 2015.

6. Ewing H. A practical guide to intervention in health and social services with pregnant and postpartum addicts and alcoholics: theoretical framework, brief screening tool, key interview questions, and strategies for referral to recovery resources. Martinez: The Born Free Project, Contra Costa County Department of Health Services; 1990.

7. Montgomery D, Plate C, Alder SC, Jones M, Jones J, Christensen RD. Testing for fetal exposure to illicit drugs using umbilical cord tissue vs meconium. J Perinatol. 2006;26(1):11–4.

8. Montgomery DP, Plate CA, Jones M, Jones J, Rios R, Lambert DK, Schumtz N, Wiedmeier SE, Burnett J, Ail S, Brandel D, Maichuck G, Durham CA, Henry E, Christensen RD. Using umbilical cord tissue to detect fetal exposure to illicit drugs: a multicentered study in Utah and New Jersey. J Perinatol. 2008;28(11):750–3. Epub 2008 Jul 3.

9. Stitely ML, Calhoun BC, Maxwell S, Nerhood R, Chaffin D. Prevalence of drug use in pregnant West Virginia patients. W V Med J. 2010;105:48–52.

10. Baxter FR, Nerhood R, Chaffin D. Characterization of babies discharged from Cabell Huntington Hospital during the calendar year 2005 with the diagnoses of neonatal abstinence syndrome. W V Med J. 2009;105(2):16–21.

11. Hensel S, Seybold D, Lewis T, Burgess D, Casto A, Calhoun BC. Substance abuse in pregnancy: role of universal urine drug screening and addiction therapy in West Virginia. Poster presentation in 16th World Congress on Controversies in Obstetrics, Gynecology, and Infertility (COGI), Singapore, 19–22 July 2012.

12. Rementeria JL, Nunag NN. Narcotic withdrawal in pregnancy. Am J Obstet Gynecol. 1973;116:1152–6.

13. Finnegan JP. Treatment issues for opioid dependent women during the perinatal period. J Psychoactive Drugs. 1991;23: 191–202.

14. Jarvis MAE, Schnoll SH. Methadone maintenance and withdrawal in pregnant opioid addicts. In: Chiang CN, Finnegan LP, editors. Medication development for the treatment of pregnant addicts and their infants. Washington, DC: US Department of Health and Human Services; 1994. p. 58–77. NIDA Monograph 149.

15. Dashe JS, Jackson GL, Olscher DA, Zane EH, Wendel GD. Opioid detoxification in pregnancy. Obstet Gynecol. 1998;92: 854–8.
16. Luty J, Nikolaou V, Bearn J. Is opiate detoxification unsafe in pregnancy? J Subst Abuse Treat. 2003;24:363–7.
17. Stewart RD, Nelson DB, Adhikari EH, McIntire DD, Roberts SW, Dashe JS, Sheffield JS. The obstetrical and neonatal impact of maternal opioid detoxification in pregnancy. Am J Obstet Gynecol. 2013;209:267.e1–5.
18. Hensel S, Seybold D, Lewis T, Burgess D, Casto A, Barnes A, Calhoun BC. Substance abuse in pregnancy: role of universal urine drug screening and outpatient addiction therapy in West Virginia. Poster presentation in 62nd annual meeting of Society for Reproductive Investigation (SGR), San Francisco, 26–28 March 2015.
19. Hoegerman G, Schnoll SH. Methadone maintenance and withdrawal in pregnant opioid addicts. Clin Perinatol. 1991;18: 51–76.
20. Briggs GG, Freeman RK, Yaffee SJ. Drugs in pregnancy and lactation. Baltimore: Williams and Wilkins; 1994. p. 557–8.
21. Cooper JR, Altman F, Brown BS, Czechowicz D, editors. Research on the treatment of narcotic addiction: state of the art. (NIDA Research Monograph 83-1201). Rockville: US Department of Health and Human Services; 1983.
22. Andres RL, Jones KL. Social and illicit drug use in pregnancy. In: Creasy RK, Resnick R, editors. Maternal-fetal medicine. Philadelphia: Saunders; 1994. p. 191–2.
23. Winklbaur B, Kopf N, Ebner N, Jung E, Thau K, Fischer G. Treating pregnant women dependent on opioids is not the same as treating pregnancy and opioid dependence: a knowledge synthesis for better treatment for women and neonates. Addiction. 2008;103:1429–40.
24. Chutuape MA, Jasinski DR, Fingerhood MI, Stitzer ML. One, three, and six month outcomes following brief inpatient opioid detoxification. Am J Drug Alcohol Abuse. 2001;27:19–44.
25. Gossop M, Green L, Phillips G, Bradley B. Lapse, relapse, and survival among opiate addicts immediately after treatment: a prospective follow-up study. Br J Psychiatry. 1989;154:348–53.
26. Silsby H, Tennat FS. Short-term, ambulatory detoxification of opiate addicts using methadone. Int J Addict. 1974;9:167–70.
27. Jones HE, Johnson RE, Jasinski DR, O'Grady KE, Chisholm CA, Choo RE, Crocetti M, Dudas R, Harrow C, Huestis MA,

Jansson LM, Lantz M, Lester BM, Milio L. Buprenorphine versus methadone in the treatment of pregnant opioid-dependent patients: effects on the neonatal abstinence syndrome. Drug Alcohol Depend. 2004;79:1–10.

28. Rothman KJ. Causes. Am J Epidemiol. 1976;104:587–92.

29. Zierler S, Rothman KJ. Congenital heart disease in relation to maternal use of Bendectin and other drugs in early pregnancy. N Engl J Med. 1985;313:347–52.

30. Braken MB. Drug use in early pregnancy and congenital hear disease in offspring. N Engl J Med. 1986;314:1120.

31. Shaw GM, Malcoe LH, Swan SH, Cummins SK, Schulman J. Congenital cardiac anomalies and conditions during early pregnancy. Eur J Epidemiol. 1992;8:757–60.

32. Braken MB, Holford TR. Exposure to prescribed drugs in pregnancy and association with congenital malformations. Obstet Gynecol. 1981;58:336–44.

33. Jick H, Holmes LB, Hunter JR, Madson S, Stergachis A. First-trimester drug use and congenital disorders. JAMA. 1981;246:343–6.

34. Broussard CS, Rasmussen SA, Reefhuis J, Friedman JM, Jann MW, Riehle-Colarusso T, et al. Maternal treatment with opioid analgesics and risk for birth defects. National Birth Defects Prevention Study. Am J Obstet Gynecol. 2011. doi:10.1016/j.ajog.2010.12.039.

35. Center for Substance Abuse Treatment. Medication-assisted treatment for opioid addiction during pregnancy. In: SAHMSA/CSAT treatment improvement protocols. Rockville: Substance Abuse and Mental Health Services Administration; 2008. Available at www.ncbi.nlm.nih.gov/books/NBK26113.

36. Substance Abuse and Mental Health Services Administration. Behavioral health barometer: United States, 2014. HHS publication no. SMA-15-4895. Rockville: Substance Abuse and Mental Health Services Administration; 2015. p. 19.

37. Substance Abuse and Mental Health Services Administration. Behavioral health barometer: United States, 2014. HHS publication no. SMA-15-4895. Rockville: Substance Abuse and Mental Health Services Administration; 2015. p. 17.

38. Substance Abuse and Mental Health Services Administration. Behavioral health barometer: United States, 2014. HHS publication no. SMA-15-4895. Rockville: Substance Abuse and Mental Health Services Administration; 2015. p. 4.

39. Tong VT, Jones JR, Dietz PM, D'Angelo D, Bombard JM. Trends in smoking before, during, and after pregnancy—Pregnancy Risk Assessment Monitoring System (PRAMS), United States, 31 sites, 2000-2005. MMWR Surveill Summ. 2009;58:1–31.
40. Jaddoe VWV, Verburg BO, de Ridder MAJ, Hofman A, Mackenbach JP, Moll HA, Steegers EAP, Witteman JCM, et al. Maternal smoking and fetal growth characteristics in different periods of pregnancy. The generation R study. Am J Epidemiol. 2007;165:1207–15.
41. Ingvarsson RF, Bjarnason AO, Dagbjartsson A, Hardardottir H, Haraldsson A, Thorkelsson T, et al. The effects of smoking in pregnancy on factors influencing fetal growth. Acta Paediatr. 2007;96:383–6.
42. Okah FA, Hoff GL, Dew P, Cai J, et al. Cumulative and residual risks of small for gestational age neonates after changing pregnancy-smoking behaviors. Am J Perinatol. 2007;24:191–6.
43. Villalbi JR, Salvador J, Cano-Serral G, Rodriguez-Sanz MC, Borrell C. Maternal smoking, social class and outcomes of pregnancy. Paediatr Perinat Epidemiol. 2007;21:441–7.
44. Burns L, Mattick RP, Wallace C. Smoking patterns and outcomes in a population of pregnant women and other substance use disorders. Nicotine Tob Res. 2008;10:969–74.
45. McCowan LM, Dekker GA, Chan EL, Stewart A, et al. Spontaneous preterm birth and small for gestational age infants in women who stop smoking early in pregnancy: prospective cohort study. BMJ. 2009;338:b1081.
46. Uncu Y, Ozcakir A, Ecran I, Bilgel N, Uncu G. Pregnant women quit smoking: what about fathers? Survey study in Bursa Region, Turkey. Croat Med J. 2005;46:832–7.
47. Salihu HM, Aliyu MH, Pierre-Louis BJ, Alexander GR. Levels of excess infant deaths attributable to maternal smoking during pregnancy in the United States. Matern Child Health J. 2003; 7:219–27.
48. Jensen MS, Toft G, Thulstrup AM, Bonde JP, Olsen J, et al. Cryptorchidism according to maternal gestational smoking. Epidemiology. 2007;18(2):220–5.
49. Honein MA, Rasmussen SA, Reefhuis J, Romitti PA, Lammer EJ, Sun L, Correa A, et al. Maternal smoking and environmental tobacco smoke exposure and the risk of orofacial clefts. Epidemiology. 2007;18(2):226–33.
50. Schmid JM, Kuehni CE, Strippoli MPF, Roiha HL, Pavlovic R, Latzin P, Gallati S, Kraemer R, Dahinden C, Frey U, on behalf of

the Swiss Pediatric Respiratory Research Group, et al. Maternal tobacco smoking and decreased leukocytes, including dendritic cells, in neonates. Pediatr Res. 2007;61(4):462–6.

51. Goksor EA, et al. The impact of pre- and post-natal smoke exposure on future asthma and bronchial hyper-responsiveness. Acta Paediatr. 2007;96:1030–5.

52. Noakes PS, Thomas R, Lane C, Mori TA, Barden AE, Devadason SG, Prescott SL, et al. Association of maternal smoking with increased infant oxidative stress at 3 months of age. Thorax. 2007;62:714–7.

53. Ananth CV, Cnattingius S, et al. Influence of maternal smoking on placental abruption in successive pregnancies: a population-based prospective cohort study in Sweden. Am J Epidemiol. 2007;166:289–95.

54. Hogberg L, Cnattingius S, et al. The influence of maternal smoking habits on the risk of subsequent stillbirth: is there a causal relation? BJOG. 2007;114:699–704.

55. Meeker JD, Missmer SA, Vitonis AF, Cramer DW, Hauser R, et al. Risk of spontaneous abortion in women with childhood exposure to parental cigarette smoke. Am J Epidemiol. 2007; 166:571–5.

56. Goodwin RD, Keyes K, Simuro N, et al. Mental disorders and nicotine dependence among pregnant women in the United States. Obstet Gynecol. 2007;109:875–83.

57. Indredavik MS, Brubakk A, Romundstad P, Vik T, et al. Prenatal smoking exposure and psychiatric symptoms in adolescence. Acta Paediatr. 2007;96:377–82.

58. Nigg JT, Breslau N, et al. Prenatal smoking exposure, low birth weight, and disruptive behavior disorders. J Am Acad Child Adolesc Psychiatry. 2007;46(3):362–9.

59. Roza SJ, Verburg BO, Jaddoe VWV, Hofman A, Mackenbach JP, Steegers EAP, Witteman JCM, Verhulst FC, Tiemeier H, et al. Effects of maternal smoking in pregnancy on prenatal brain development. The General R Study. Eur J Neurosci. 2007;25: 611–7.

60. Lambe M, Hultman C, Torrang A, Maccabe J, Cnattingius S. Maternal smoking during pregnancy and school performance at age 16. Epidemiology. 2006;17:524–30.

61. Lumley J, Oliver SS, Chamberlain C, Oakley L. Interventions for promoting smoking cessation during pregnancy (Review). The Cochrane Collaboration. 2008(1).

62. Mainous AG, Hueston WJ. The effect of smoking cessation during pregnancy on preterm delivery and low birthweight. J Fam Pract. 1994;38:262–6.

63. Bernstein IM, Mongeon JA, Badger GJ, Solomon L, Heil SH, Higgins ST. Maternal smoking and its association with birth weight. Obstet Gynecol. 2005;106:986–91.

64. Horta BL, Victora CG, Menezes AM, Halpern R, Barros FC. Low birthweight, preterm births and intrauterine growth retardation in relation to maternal smoking. Paediatr Perinat Epidemiol. 1997;11:140–51.

65. Gnann H, Engelman C, Skopp G, Winkler M, Auwarter V, Dresen S, et al. Identification of 48 homologues of phosphatidyl-ethanol in blood by LC-ESI-MS/MS. Anal Bioanal Chem. 2010;396:2415–23.

66. Gunnarson T, Karlsson A, Hansson P, Johnson G, Alling C, Odham G. Determination of phosphatidylethanol in blood from alcoholic males using high-performance liquid chromatography and evaporative light scattering or electrospray mass spectrometric detection. J Chromatogr B Biomed Sci Appl. 1998;705: 243–9.

67. Helander A, Zheng Y. Molecular species of the alcohol biomarker phosphatidylethanol in human blood measured by LC-MS. Clin Chem. 2009;55:1395–405.

68. Kwak HS, Han JY, Ahn HK, Kim MH, Ryu HM, Kim MY, et al. Blood levels of phosphatidylethanol in pregnant women reporting positive alcohol ingestion, measured by an improved LC-MS/MS analytical method. Clin Toxicol. 2012;50:886–91.

69. Kwak HS, Han JY, Choi JS, Ahn HK, Ryu HM, Chung HJ, Cho DH, Shin CY, Velazqueza-Armenta EY, Nava-Ocampo AA. Characterization of phosphatidylethanol blood concentrations for screening alcohol consumption in early pregnancy. Clin Toxicol. 2014;52:25–31.

70. Varga A, Hansson P, Johnson G, Alling C. Normalization rate and cellular localization of phosphatidylethanol in whole blood from chronic alcoholics. Clin Chim Acta. 2000;299:141–50.

71. Gnann H, Weinmann W, Thierauf A. Formation of phosphatidyl-ethanol and its subsequent elimination during an extensive drinking experiment over 5 days. Alcohol Clin Exp Res. 2012; 36:1507–11.

72. Yamamoto Y, Yamamoto K, Fukui Y, Kurishita A. Teratogenic effects of metamphetamine in mice. Nihon Hoigaku Zasshi. 1992;46:126–31.

73. Colado ML, O'Shea E, Granados R, Misra A, Murray TK, et al. A study of the neurotoxic effect of MDMA ('ecstasy') on 5-HT neurones in the brains of mothers and neonates following administration of the drug during pregnancy. Br J Pharmacol. 1997;121:827–33.

74. He N, Lidow MS. Cerebral cortical abnormalities seen in non-human primate model of prenatal cocaine exposure are not related to vasoconstriction. Neurotoxicology. 2004;25:419–32.

75. Plessinger MA. Prenatal exposure to amphetamines. Risks and adverse outcomes in pregnancy. Obstet Gynecol Clin North Am. 1998;25:119–38.

76. Nora JJ, Vargo TA, Nora AH, Love KE, McNamara DG. Dexamphetamine: a possible environmental trigger in cardio-vascular malformations. Lancet. 1970;1:1290–1.

77. Bays J. Fetal vascular disruption with prenatal exposure to cocaine or metamphetamine. Pediatrics. 1994;87:416–8.

78. Lipshultz SE, Frassiac JJ, Orav EJ. Cardiovascular abnormalities in infants prenatally exposed to cocaine. J Pediatr. 1991;118:44–51.

79. Srisurapanont M, Jarusuraisin N, Kittirattanapaiboon P. Treatment for amphetamine dependence and abuse. Cochrane Database Syst Rev. 2001,(4):CD003022.

80. Trezza V, Campolongo P, Cassano T, et al. Effects of perinatal exposure to delta-9-tetrahydrocannabinol on the emotional reactivity of the offspring: a longitudinal behavioral study in Wistar rats. Psychopharmacology (Berl). 2008;198(4):529–37.

81. Fried PA, Makin JE. Neonatal behavioral correlates of prenatal exposure to marijuana, cigarettes, and alcohol in a low risk population. Neurotoxicol Teratol. 1987;9:1–7.

82. de Moraes Barros MC, Guinsburg R, de Araujo Peres C, Mitsuhiro S, Chalem E, Laranjeira RR. Neurobehavioral profile of healthy full-term newborn infants of adolescent mothers. Early Hum Dev. 2008;84:281–7.

83. Goldschmidt L, Day NL, Richardson GA. Effects of prenatal marijuana exposure on child behavior problems at age 10. Neurotoxicol Teratol. 2000;22(3):325–36.

84. Richardson GA, Ryan C, Willford J, Day NL, Goldschmidt L. Prenatal alcohol and marijuana exposure: effects on neuropsy-chological outcomes at 10 years. Neurotoxicol Teratol. 2002;4(3):309–20.

85. Schempf AH, Strobino DM. Illicit drug use and adverse birth outcomes: is it drugs or context? J Urban Health. 2008;85(6):858–73.

86. Webster WS, Brown-Woodman PD. Cocaine as a cause for congenital malformations of vascular origin: experimental evidence in the rat. Teratology. 1990;41:689–97.
87. Frank DA, Augustyn M, Knight WG, et al. Growth, development, and behavior in early childhood following prenatal cocaine exposure: a systematic review. JAMA. 2001;285:1613.
88. Substance Abuse and Mental Health Services Administration. Results from the 2011 National Survey on Drug Use and Health: mental health findings. 2012.
89. Kessler RC, McGonagle KA, Zhao S, Nelson CB, Hughes M, Eshleman S, Wittchen HU, Kendler KS. Lifetime and 12-month prevalence of DSM-III-R psychiatric disorders in the United States. Results from the National Comorbidity Survey. Arch Gen Psychiatry. 1994;51(1):8–19. doi:10.1001/archpsyc.51.1.8.
90. Regier DA, Farmer ME, Rae DS, Locke BZ, Keith SJ, Judd LL, Goodwin FK. Comorbidity of mental disorders with alcohol and other drug abuse. Results from the Epidemiologic Catchment Area (ECA) Study. JAMA. 1990;264(19):2511–8. doi:10.1001/jama.264.19.2511.
91. Drake RE, Wallach MA. Moderate drinking among people with severe mental illness. Hosp Community Psychiatry. 1993;44(8):780–2.
92. Dutra L, Statthopoulou G, Basden SL, Leyro TM, Powers MB, Otto MW. A meta-analytic review of psychosocial interventions for substance use disorders. Am J Psychiatry. 2008;165:179–87.
93. Moran P, Madgula RM, Gilvarry E, Findlay M. Substance misuse during pregnancy: its effects and treatment. Fetal Maternal Med Rev. 2009;20:1–16.

Chapter 2
Physiology of Nicotine

Paul Dietz

Introduction

Nicotine is a stimulating drug used both medically and recreationally in the United States. It is one of the most addictive agents known to science and a major contributing factor to the addictive properties of tobacco use. The nicotine content of popular American-brand cigarettes has slowly increased over the years, and one study found that there was an average increase of 1.78 % per year between the years of 1998 and 2005 [1].

Background

First introduced to Western culture in Europe in 1559, nicotine is named after the tobacco plant *Nicotiana tabacum*, which received its name from the French ambassador to Portugal, Jean Nicot de Villemain. In 1560, de Villemain, sent tobacco and seeds to Paris as a gift to French King Henry II,

P. Dietz, MD, FACOG (✉)
Department of Obstetrics and Gynecology, Charleston Area
Women's Medicine Center, Medical Center, Charleston, WV, USA
e-mail: paul.dietz@camc.org

© Springer International Publishing Switzerland 2016
B.C. Calhoun, T. Lewis (eds.), *Tobacco Cessation and
Substance Abuse Treatment in Women's Healthcare*,
DOI 10.1007/978-3-319-26710-4_2

who advocated its medicinal use. Luis de Gois, a Portuguese colonist from Sao Paulo, brought the tobacco and seeds to de Villemain from Brazil. Tobacco use was believed to protect against illness, most notably the plague [2].

After its introduction, tobacco was not only smoked recreationally, but also used as an insecticide. After World War II, over 2500 tons of nicotine insecticide were used around the world, but its use has significantly declined since the 1980s with the availability of other agents being cheaper and less harmful to mammals [3]. The United States currently prohibits the use of nicotine as a pesticide for organic farming [4, 5]. The EPA received a request in 2008 to cancel the registration of the last nicotine pesticide in the United States [6]. This request was formally granted and since January 2014, this pesticide has not been available for sale [7].

Nicotine was first isolated from the tobacco plant in 1828 by physician Wilhelm Heinrich Posselt and chemist Karl Ludwig Reimann in Germany and was considered a poison [8, 9]. The empirical chemical formula was described by Melsens in 1843 and its structure discovered by Adolf Pinner and Richard Wolffenstein in 1893 [9, 10]. It was first synthesized in 1904 by Amé Pictet and A. Rotschy [10].

Pharmacology

Nicotine is powerful parasympathomimetic alkaloid found in the nightshade family of plants (*Solanaceae*) and considered a stimulant drug [11]. It is produced in the roots of and accumulates in the leaves of the nightshade family of plants. Specifically, nicotine is found in the leaves of *Nicotiana tabacum* and *Nicotiana rustica* in amounts near 15 %, as well as in *Duboisia hopwoodii* and *Asclepias syriaca* [12].

Nicotine is a hygroscopic, colorless oily liquid that is readily soluble in alcohol, ether or light petroleum. It is miscible with water in its base form between 60 and 210 °C. As a nitrogenous base, nicotine forms salts with acids that are usually solid and water soluble. Its flash point is 95 °C and its auto-ignition temperature is 244 °C [13].

Nicotine is optically active, having two enantiomeric forms. The naturally occurring form of nicotine is levorotatory with a specific rotation of $[\alpha]_D = -166.4°$ ((−)-nicotine). The dextrorotatory form, (+)-nicotine is physiologically less active than (−)-nicotine. (−)-nicotine is more toxic than (+)-nicotine [14]. The salts of (+)-nicotine are usually dextrorotatory. The hydrochloride and sulphate salts become optically inactive if heated in a closed vessel above 180 °C. On exposure to ultraviolet light or various oxidizing agents, nicotine is converted to nicotine oxide, nicotinic acid (vitamin B3), and methylamine [15].

As nicotine enters the body, it is distributed quickly through the bloodstream and crosses the blood–brain barrier reaching the brain within 10–20 s after inhalation [16]. The elimination half-life of nicotine in the body is around 2 h [17].

The amount of nicotine absorbed by the body from smoking can depend on many factors, including the types of tobacco, whether the smoke is inhaled, and whether a filter is used. However, it has been found that the nicotine yield of individual products has only a small effect (4.4 %) on the blood concentration of nicotine [18], suggesting "the assumed health advantage of switching to lower-tar and lower-nicotine cigarettes may be largely offset by the tendency of smokers to compensate by increasing inhalation."

Nicotine acts on nicotinic acetylcholine receptors, specifically the α3β4 ganglion type nicotinic receptor, present in the autonomic ganglia and adrenal medulla, and a central nervous system (CNS) α4β2 nicotinic receptor. In small concentrations, nicotine increases the activity of these cholinergic receptors and indirectly on a variety of other neurotransmitters such as dopamine.

Nicotine is metabolized in the liver by cytochrome P450 enzymes (mostly CYP2A6, and also by CYP2B6). A major metabolite is cotinine. Other primary metabolites include nicotine N'-oxide, nornicotine, nicotine isomethonium ion, 2-hydroxynicotine, and nicotine glucuronide [19]. Under some conditions, other substances may be formed such as myosmine [20]. Glucuronidation and oxidative metabolism of nicotine to cotinine are both inhibited by menthol, an additive to mentholated cigarettes, thus increasing the half-life of nicotine in vivo [21].

Nicotine can be quantified in blood, plasma, or urine to confirm a diagnosis of poisoning or to facilitate a medicolegal death investigation. Urinary or salivary cotinine concentrations are frequently measured for the purposes of pre-employment and health insurance medical screening programs. Careful interpretation of results is important, since passive exposure to cigarette smoke can result in significant accumulation of nicotine, followed by the appearance of its metabolites in various body fluids [22, 23]. Nicotine use is not regulated in competitive sports programs [24].

Physical and Chemical Properties

Nicotine is a hygroscopic, colorless oily liquid that is readily soluble in alcohol, ether or light petroleum. It is miscible with water in its base form between 60 and 210 °C. As a nitrogenous base, nicotine forms salts with acids that are usually solid and water soluble. Its flash point is 95 °C and its auto-ignition temperature is 244 °C [13]. Nicotine is readily volatile (vapor pressure 5.5 Pa at 25 °C) and dibasic ($K_{b1} = 1 \times 10^{-6}$, $K_{b2} = 1 \times 10^{-11}$) [12].

Nicotine is a natural product of tobacco, occurring in the leaves in a range of 0.5–7.5 % depending on variety [25]. Nicotine also naturally occurs in smaller amounts in plants from the family *Solanaceae* (such as potatoes, tomatoes, and eggplant) [26]. The biosynthetic pathway of nicotine involves a coupling reaction between the two cyclic structures that compose nicotine. Metabolic studies show that the pyridine ring of nicotine is derived from niacin (nicotinic acid) while the pyrrolidone is derived from *N*-methyl-Δ^1-pyrrollidium cation [27, 28]. Biosynthesis of the two component structures proceeds via two independent syntheses, the NAD pathway for niacin and the tropane pathway for *N*-methyl-Δ^1-pyrrollidium cation.

The NAD pathway in the genus *nicotiana* begins with the oxidation of aspartic acid into α-imino succinate by aspartate oxidase. This is followed by a condensation with glyceraldehyde-3-phosphate and a cyclization catalyzed by quinolinate synthase to give quinolinic acid. Quinolinic acid then reacts with phosphoribosyl pyrophosphate catalyzed by quinolinic acid phosphoribosyl transferase to form niacin mononucleotide. The reaction now proceeds via the NAD salvage cycle to produce niacin via the conversion of nicotinamide by the enzyme nicotinamidase.

The N-methyl-Δ^1-pyrrollidium cation used in the synthesis of nicotine is an intermediate in the synthesis of tropane-derived alkaloids. Biosynthesis begins with decarboxylation of ornithine by ornithine decarboxylase to produce putrescine. Putrescine is then converted into N-methyl putrescine via methylation by SAM catalyzed by putrescine N-methyltransferase. N-methylputrescine then undergoes deamination into 4-methyl-aminobutanal by the N-methylputrescine oxidase enzyme, 4-methylaminobutanal then spontaneously cyclize into N-methyl-Δ^1-pyrrollidium cation.

The final step in the synthesis of nicotine is the coupling between N-methyl-Δ^1-pyrrollidium cation and niacin. Although studies conclude some form of coupling between the two component structures, the definite process and mechanism remains undetermined. The current agreed theory involves the conversion of niacin into 2,5-dihydropyridine through 3,6-dihydronicotinic acid. The 2,5-dihydropyridine intermediate would then react with N-methyl-Δ^1-pyrrollidium cation to form enantiomerically pure (−)-nicotine [29].

Research

While acute/initial nicotine intake causes activation of nicotine receptors, chronic low doses of nicotine use leads to desensitization of nicotine receptors (due to the development of tolerance) and results in an antidepressant effect, with research showing low-dose nicotine patches being an effective treatment of major depressive disorder in non-smokers [30]. However, the original research concluded that: "Nicotine patches produced short-term improvement of depression with minor side effects. Because of nicotine's high risk to health, nicotine patches are not recommended for clinical use in depression" [31].

Though tobacco smoking is associated with an increased risk of Alzheimer's disease [32], there is evidence that nicotine itself has the potential to prevent and treat Alzheimer's disease [33].

Research into nicotine's most predominant metabolite, cotinine, suggests that some, if not most, of nicotine's psychoactive effects may actually be mediated by complex interactions with cotinine, or perhaps even by cotinine alone rather than strictly by nicotine as conventionally thought [34, 35].

Little research is available in humans but animal research suggests there is potential benefit from nicotine in Parkinson's disease [36]. There is tentative evidence that nicotinamides may improve depression [37].

References

1. Connolly GN, Alpert HR, Wayne GF, Koh H. Trends in nicotine yield in smoke and its relationship with design characteristics among popular US cigarette brands, 1997-2005. Tob Control. 2007;16(5):e5.
2. Ujváry I. Nicotine and other insecticidal alkaloids. In: Yamamoto I, Casida J, editors. Nicotinoid insecticides and the nicotinic acetylcholine receptor. Tokyo: Springer; 1999. p. 29–69.
3. Rang HP, et al. Rang and Dale's pharmacology. 6th ed. Amsterdam: Elsevier; 2007. p. 598.
4. US Code of Federal Regulations. 7 CFR 205.602—Nonsynthetic substances prohibited for use in organic crop production.
5. Staff, IFOAM. Criticisms and frequent misconceptions about organic agriculture: the counter-arguments: misconception number.
6. USEPA. Nicotine; notice of receipt of request to voluntarily cancel a pesticide registration. Federal Register: 64320–64322; 29 Oct 2008. Retrieved 8 April 2012.

7. USEPA. Nicotine; product cancellation order. Federal Register: 26695–26696; 3 June 2009. Retrieved 8 April 2012.
8. Posselt W, Reimann L. Chemische Untersuchung des Tabaks und Darstellung eines eigenthümlich wirksamen Prinzips dieser Pflanze [Chemical investigation of tobacco and preparation of a characteristically active constituent of this plant]. Magazin für Pharmacie (in German). 1828;6(24):138–61.
9. Henningfield JE, Zeller M. Nicotine psychopharmacology research contributions to United States and global tobacco regulation: a look back and a look forward. Psychopharmacology (Berl). 2006;184(3–4):286–91.
10. Pictet A, Rotschy A. Synthese des Nicotins. Berichte der deutschen chemischen Gesellschaft. 1904;37(2):1225–35.
11. Nicotinic acetylcholine receptors: introduction. IUPHAR Database. International Union of Basic and Clinical Pharmacology. Retrieved 1 Sept 2014.
12. Metcalf RL. Insect control. In: Ullmann's encyclopedia of industrial chemistry. 7th ed. New York: Wiley; 2007. p. 9.
13. Material safety data sheet L-nicotine MSDS.
14. Gause GF. Chapter V: Analysis of various biological processes by the study of the differential action of optical isomers. In: Luyet BJ, editor. Optical activity and living matter. A series of monographs on general physiology 2. Normandy: Biodynamica; 1941.
15. http://library.sciencemadness.org/library/books/the_plant_alkaloids.pdf.
16. Le Houezec J. Role of nicotine pharmacokinetics in nicotine addiction and nicotine replacement therapy: a review. Int J Tuberc Lung Dis. 2003;7(9):811–9.
17. Benowitz NL, Jacob P, Jones RT, Rosenberg J. Interindividual variability in the metabolism and cardiovascular effects of nicotine in man. J Pharmacol Exp Ther. 1982;221(2):368–72.
18. Russell MA, Jarvis M, Iyer R, Feyerabend C. Relation of nicotine yield of cigarettes to blood nicotine concentrations in smokers. Br Med J. 1980;280(6219):972–6.
19. Hukkanen J, Jacob P, Benowitz NL. Metabolism and disposition kinetics of nicotine. Pharmacol Rev. 2005;57(1):79–115.
20. The danger of third-hand smoke. Chromatography Online 7(3).
21. Benowitz NL, Herrera B, Jacob III P. Mentholated cigarette smoking inhibits nicotine metabolism. J Pharmacol Exp Ther. 2004;310(3):1208–15.

22. Benowitz NL, Hukkanen J, Jacob P. Nicotine psychopharmacology. Handbook of experimental pharmacology. Handb Exp Pharmacol. 2009;192(192):29–60.

23. Baselt RC. Disposition of toxic drugs and chemicals in man. 10th ed. Seal Beach: Biomedical Publications; 2014. p. 1452–6.

24. Mündel T, Jones DA. Effect of transdermal nicotine administration on exercise endurance in men. Exp Physiol. 2006;91(4):705–13.

25. Tobacco (leaf tobacco). Transportation Information Service.

26. Domino EF, Hornbach E, Demana T. The nicotine content of common vegetables. N Engl J Med. 1993;329:437.

27. Lamberts BL, Dewey LJ, Byerrum RU. Ornithine as a precursor for the pyrrolidine ring of nicotine. Biochim Biophys Acta. 1959;33(1):22–6.

28. Dawson RF, Christman DR, d'Adamo A, Solt ML, Wolf AP. The biosynthesis of nicotine from isotopically labeled nicotinic acids. J Am Chem Soc. 1960;82(10):2628–33.

29. Ashihara H, Crozier A, Komamine A, editors. Plant metabolism and biotechnology. Cambridge: Wiley; 2011.

30. Mineur YS, Picciotto MR. Nicotine receptors and depression: revisiting and revising the cholinergic hypothesis. Trends Pharmacol Sci. 2010;31(12):580–6.

31. Salín-Pascual RJ, Rosas M, Jimenez-Genchi A, Rivera-Meza BL, Delgado-Parra V. Antidepressant effect of transdermal nicotine patches in nonsmoking patients with major depression. J Clin Psychiatry. 1996;59(9):387–9.

32. Peters R, Poulter R, Warner J, Beckett N, Burch L, Bulpitt C. Smoking, dementia and cognitive decline in the elderly, a systematic review. BMC Geriatr. 2008;8:36.

33. Henningfield JE, Zeller M. Nicotine psychopharmacology: policy and regulatory. Handbook experimental pharmacology. Handb Exp Pharmacol. 2009;192(192):511–34.

34. Grizzell JA, Echeverria V. New insights into the mechanisms of action of cotinine and its distinctive effects from nicotine. Neurochem Res. 2015;40:2032–46.

35. Crooks PA, Dwoskin LP. Contribution of CNS nicotine metabolites to the neuropharmacological effects of nicotine and tobacco smoking. Biochem Pharmacol. 1997;1(54):743–53.

36. Barreto GE, Iarkov A, Moran VE. Beneficial effects of nicotine, cotinine and its metabolites as potential agents for Parkinson's disease. Front Aging Neurosci. 2015;9(6):340.

37. http://www.sciencedaily.com/releases/2006/09/060912225448.htm. www.sciencedaily.com.

Chapter 3
Physiology of EtOH, Opiate, Hypnotics, and Stimulants Receptors

Byron C. Calhoun

Pharmacokinetics

Pharmacokinetics involves the amount of time it takes for drugs to develop concentrations in blood and tissue (brain). Drug concentrations in blood and other tissues are influenced the absorption, distribution, metabolism, and elimination of the drug. A drug's pharmacologic effects are directly related to the amount of the free or unbound drug concentration at its sit of action.

Absorption entails the process of the drug movement from the site of drug delivery to the site of action. Psychoactive drugs may be taken orally (ethanol, amphetamine, barbiturates, opiates), intranasally (glue, solvents, amyl nitrate, cocaine, heroin), via smoking (nicotine, marijuana, freebase cocaine), intravenously (heroin, cocaine, methamphetamine), transdermally (fentanyl and nicotine patches), and subcutaneous injection. Drug concentrations vary by time over the various routes of administration. The more rapidly the psychoactive drug is delivered to the site of action in the brain,

B.C. Calhoun, MD, FACOG, FACS, FASAM, MBA (✉)
Department of Obstetrics and Gynecology, West Virginia
University-Charleston, Charleston, WV, USA
e-mail: Byron.calhoun@camc.org

© Springer International Publishing Switzerland 2016   33
B.C. Calhoun, T. Lewis (eds.), *Tobacco Cessation and
Substance Abuse Treatment in Women's Healthcare*,
DOI 10.1007/978-3-319-26710-4_3

the greater is its mood-altering and reinforcing effects. The most rapid achieved and highest peak concentrations are achieved from the pulmonary and intravenous routes.

Bioavailability consists of the fraction of unchanged drug that reaches the systemic circulation after administration by various routes. The bioavailability factor (F) adjusts for the portion of administered dose that is able to enter the bloodstream in unchanged form. For example, the amount of drug available after intravenous administration is equal to 100 % ($F=1.0$). Bioavailability depends on the drug's site-specific membrane permeability, activity of the receptors, and the first-pass metabolism. First-pass metabolism represents the metabolism that takes place before the drug reaches the bloodstream and occurs most completely for lipid-soluble drugs like morphine, methylphenidate, and desipramine. This effect significantly reduces bioavailability of the drugs. An example is morphine which requires double the dose when administered orally compared to intravenous administration. First-pass metabolism is not important for intravenous, sublingual, intramuscular, subcutaneous, and transdermal routes due to the entry directly into the blood stream.

Oral administration absorption is influenced by several phenomena: pharmaceutical properties of the drug, the pH of the gastric contents, gastric emptying time (distribution to small intestines for absorption), intestinal transit time (i.e., drugs absorbed in small intestine absorb faster with faster transit time), integrity of intestinal epithelium, and the presence of food [1]. Smoked and inhaled drugs completely bypass the venous system and have most rapid rate of delivery. Absorption of the inhaled drugs depends on the physical characteristics of the drug, especially the drugs' volatility, particle size, and lipid solubility [2]. Drugs that are inhaled have essentially unlimited access to the vascularity through the interface of the surface of the alveoli with the central pulmonary vessels. Due to the rapid flow of the cardiac output, smoked, and freebase drugs rapidly enter the brain.

All drugs must pass through cell membranes for absorption. Passive diffusion favors lipid-soluble and uncharged molecules. Others have decreased absorption due to the effects of the reverse transporter of P-glycoprotein. This reverse transporter actually pumps drugs from the gut epithelium back into the gut itself thereby decreasing absorption. Other food and drug interactions change the first-pass phenomenon. Grapefruit juice and other foods that either inhibit or induce intestinal wall CY3A4 or P-glycoprotein may lead to altered bioavailability of drugs that are substrates for this cytochrome [3, 4]. The class of monoamine oxidase inhibitors (MAOIs) such as phenelzine and tranylcypromine inhibit monoamine oxidase-A in the intestinal wall and liver. This inhibition diminishes the first-pass metabolism of tyramine that is present in cheese, wines, and various other foods. When tyramine, an indirect acting sympathomimetic amine, reaches the blood stream, it can produce increased release of norepinephrine from the sympathetic postganglionic neurons which may result in severe pressor response and hypertensive crisis.

Increasing gastric emptying time may help to increase a more rapid drug effect without any change in bioavailability. Gastric emptying may be increased by drinking at least 200 mL of water and staying upright. Delay of gastric emptying, and, hence later and lower peaks of drug concentrations, include food, heavy exercise, recumbency, and drugs that slow gastric emptying (narcotics and anticholinergic drugs).

Distribution

Distribution is influenced b organ perfusion, organ size, binding of the drugs within the blood and tissues, and permeability of the tissue membranes [5]. The majority of psychoactive drugs enter the brain because of high lipid solubility. The blood–brain barrier restricts entry by non-lipid-soluble drugs into the brain by diffusion. The brain's capillaries prevent the entry of molecules less than 25,000 Da due to the lack of fenestrations in the capillaries. Without fenestrations, the drugs must pass through the two membranes of the endothelial cells by passive diffusion. This barrier limits access by numerous drugs to the brain, spinal cord, and all areas of the subarachnoid membrane, except the floor of the hypothalamus.

Some compounds have active transport systems. These active transport systems enable glucose, amino acids, amines, purines, nucleosides, and organic acids to enter the brain [6]. The distribution of drugs to all parts of the body consists of the volume of distribution (V_d). The volume does consist of a quantifiable physical equivalent, but rather, the amount of serum, plasma, or blood that would be required for all the drug in the body. V_d can be thought of the amount of drug in the body (D = dose) divided by the concentration of drug (C) in the plasma. Drugs with a small volume of distribution are found mostly in the intravascular space of about 5 L. Drugs that are tightly bound to plasma proteins, or have a high molecular weight (large proteins, dextran, and others) may have a volume of distribution up to 50,000 L.

Protein-binding affects the free and active drug concentration. Proteins generally have characteristics of capacity (amount of bind space) and affinity (tightness of binding). For example, albumin is a high-capacity, low-affinity-binding protein unlike a specific transport protein such as transcortin which is a low capacity, high-affinity protein. Acidic drugs usually bind to albumin, the most abundant plasma protein. Examples include barbiturates, benzodiazepines, and phenytoin. Basic drugs like methadone bind to alpha$_1$-acid glycoprotein, and others such as amitriptyline and nortriptyline bind to lipoproteins. There are binding sites that are competitive, and drugs with a higher binding site affinity can displace a drug with a lower binding site affinity. It may also be stereospecific (for one stereoisomer of a compound). Drugs that are greater than 90 % bound are considered highly protein bound, and reduced protein binding for highly protein bound drugs can lead to large increases in drug effect.

The rate of blood flow delivered to specific organs and tissues affects drug distribution. Well-perfused tissues may receive large quantities of drug provided that the drug can cross the membranes or other cell barriers between the plasma and tissue. In contrast, poorly perfused tissues, such as fat, receive and release drug at a slow rate. This explains why concentrations of drugs may be maintained long after the concentration in plasma has begun to decrease. An example is anesthetics.

Clearance of drugs is usually described as elimination. Elimination consists of the disappearance of the parent drug and/or its active molecule from the bloodstream or body. This may occur by either metabolism and/or excretion. Excretion is removing a compound from the body without chemically altering the compound. Drugs may be excreted through urine, feces, exhaled through the lungs, or secreted in sweat or salivary glands. The term clearance (CI) represents the theoretical volume of blood or plasma that is completely cleared of a given drug over a specific period of time. Factors that determine liver clearance are hepatic blood flow, the fraction of drug that is unbound, and the drug's intrinsic clearance. If the intrinsic clearance of the unbound drug is small, then the metabolic capacity (intrinsic clearance) of the liver, rather than hepatic blood flow, becomes the major determinant of hepatic clearance. In that case, the functionality of the hepatic enzymes determines drug clearance. If the intrinsic clearance of an unbound drug is very large, blood flow to the liver becomes rate limiting. Metabolic capacity determines drug clearance in most cases.

The majority of drugs have first-order elimination kinetics: the fraction or percentage of the total amount of drug present is removed at one time is constant and independent of dosage. After drug administration of a drug with first-order kinetics, concentrations of the drug show an exponential decline of drug concentration. The slope of the decay line is the elimination constant k_{el} which is the percent of drug cleared per unit time (i.e., percent/h). The half-life ($t_{1/2}$) of a drug is the amount of time it takes for a drug concentration to decrease by half. One half-life represents a 50 % change, and a 2, 3, 4, and 5 half-lives represent 75, 87.5, 93.7, and 96.8 % changes. The time to reach steady state depends upon the duration of the half-life, whereas the amount of drug in the body at steady state will depend upon the frequency of the drug administration and its dose. With drugs with dose-dependent (first-order) disposition and elimination characteristics, 5 half-lives is a reasonable estimate of the time to reach steady state for the given drug. For example, if the concentration at 2 h postdose is 100 µg/mL, and the concentration at 4 h postdose is 50 µg/mL, the $t_{1/2}$ is 2 h.

Drug metabolism is the process of chemical modification of drugs and other chemicals by the body, generally into less active and more hydrophilic compounds. These chemical modifications/reactions are generally performed by enzymatic systems, such as the cytochrome P450 enzyme system. Lipophilic drugs are generally transformed to more hydrophilic/polar products that are inactive or nontoxic, and active metabolites need to be considered when assessing a drug's activity. In certain cases, the administered drug is intentionally designed to be a pharmacologically inactive prodrug that is converted in vivo to a pharmacologically active molecule. One example is levodopa which, after crossing the blood–brain barrier, is converted in the basal ganglia to dopamine.

Drugs may be metabolized by Phase I/or Phase II reactions. Phase I reactions are nonsynthetic reactions in which the drug is chemically altered and oxidized. For example, a drug may be demethylated. Examples of Phase I reactions include the oxidation of phenobarbital, amphetamine, meperidine, and codeine by microsomal enzymes. Phase II reactions are synthetic reactions in which the drug is conjugated with another moiety, such as glucuronide or sulfate. Examples of synthetic reactions include glucuronidation of morphine and meprobamate and acetylation of clonazepam and mescaline, which produce a compounds more polar than the parent drugs in order to facilitate metabolism. Cytochrome P450 enzymes are most commonly involved and exist in the gut, liver, and brain. The gut and liver enzymes are the best studied. Oxidations can take place by cytochromic P450-dependent and cytochrome P450-independent mechanisms. Cytochrome P450-dependent oxidations include aromatic (phenytoin, amphetamine) and aliphatic (pentobarbital, meprobamate) hydroxylations, epoxidation, and oxidative dealkylation (morphine, caffeine, codeine), deamination (amphetamine), desulfurization (thiopental), and dechlorination. Cytochrome P450-independent oxidations include dehydrogenations (ethanol); azo, nitro, and carbonyl reductions (methadone, naloxone); and ester and amide hydrolysis [7].

The other family of enzymes identified in the metabolism of drugs is the CYP group. This family of enzymes is involved in the metabolism of dietary and environmental compounds and medications. These enzymes are involved in a large number of endogenous functions (as in bile acids). CYPs that metabolize drugs operate in a large and fluid substrate-binding sites contribute to the slow catalytic rates. One particular CYP (CYP3A4) is responsible for metabolizing more than 50 % of clinically prescribed drugs.

Pharmacogenetics

Pharmacogenetics represents the study of the relationship between genetic variations and drug disposition and responses. It necessarily entails the clarification of cytochrome and other drug-metabolizing enzyme polymorphisms (different enzyme genetic subtypes), the degree of expression of polymorphisms, and the functional significance of expression. Understanding polymorphisms of expression may help explain individual differences in drug response by individuals. Genetic variability in drug-metabolizing enzymes may affect drug bioavailability and clearance [8–11]. Single nucleotide polymorphisms (SNPs) may alter CYP activity. One example is CYP2D6 which metabolizes codeine to morphine is one of the best elucidated of the drug metabolic enzymes. There are 48 mutations and 50 alleles that have been identified. The genotype and enzyme activity are linked to patient ethnicity which may vary from no gene/no enzyme activity (6 % of Caucasians) to two copies of a fully active gene (36 % of Ethiopians). Individuals may be genotyped for 2D6 enzyme function with classification as poor metabolizers, intermediate metabolizers, extensive metabolizers, and ultrarapid metabolizers [12]. Poor metabolizers do not receive adequate analgesia due to the inability to metabolize codeine into its active metabolite of morphine. Ultrarapid metabolizers metabolize codeine into morphine producing rare but life-threatening morphine intoxication. Even infants of mothers who are ultrarapid metabolizers may receive morphine overdoses if breastfed after the mother receives codeine postpartum [13, 14].

Further evaluation of other enzyme subgroups have found other genetic drug interactions. CYP2B6 has an allele for the *4 allele with higher conversion of bupropion to the active and longer lasting metabolite, hydroxybupropion with subsequent toxicity. Other alleles were noted to have less enzyme present and less activity. These poor metabolizers necessitated an increase dosage to improve smoking cessation with bupropion [15]. The enzyme of CYP3A4 has several SNPs. The prediction of the activity of f CYP3A4 is complex and not directly related to the genotype [12]. Several opioids, including methadone and buprenorphine utilize the CYP3A4 enzyme pathway. Methadone is metabolized primarily by the CYP3A4 enzyme with further actions by CYP2B6, 2C19, 3A4, and CYP2D6 [4, 16]. Known inhibitors of CYP3A4 enzymes include erythromycin, diltiazem, ketoconazole, and saquinavir slow the metabolism of methadone and increase methadone levels. Inducers of CYP3A4 such as carbamazepine, phenobarbital, efavirenz, and St. John's wort speed the metabolism of methadone and decrease methadone levels. Due to these variations in effects, it is necessary to know potential interactions, make pertinent clinical observations, and tailor medication regimens and dosages to optimize therapy and minimize possible toxicities.

Genetic differences in drug metabolism may influence the risk of addiction with protective effects with individuals who experience adverse drug reactions at lower drug levels. The alleles of ADH1B2-His47Arg of alcohol dehydrogenase 1B and ALDH-Glu487Lys allele of aldehyde dehydrogenase 2 alone or together can lead to flushing, nausea, and headache as a result of the accumulation of acetaldehyde when alcohol is consumed. Either allele leads to a reduction in the risk of alcoholism, with addictive protective effects when the same person carries both alleles. Individuals of South Asian descent are apt to carry both alleles, whereas those with Jewish descent often have the Arg47 allele. Heterozygous carriers of ALDH2 Lys487 have low levels of ALDH2 enzyme activity, whereas ALDH2 Lys487/Lys487 homozygous individuals are nearly completely protected from alcoholism [17]. Further, slow nicotine metabolism by CYP2D6 seems to have a protective effect against nicotine addiction [18]. This also allows for increased ability to obtain nicotine abstinence.

Most drug metabolism occurs in the liver as well as lungs, GI tract, skin, and kidneys. Several P450 cytochromes have been shown to catalyze the metabolism of neurosteroids as well as psychoactive drugs such as neuroleptics and antidepressants. Alcohol produces a three- to fivefold increase in the level of P450 and induces CYP2C, CYP2E1, and CYP4A [19]. Brain CYP2D6 will demethylate 3,4-methylenedioxy-N-methylamphetamine (MDMA-ecstasy) creating the toxic metabolite N-methyl-a-methyldopamine. Brain CYP2D6 may also O-demethylate paramethoxyamphetamine, a synthetic psychostimulant and hallucinogen into the toxic compound 4-hydroxyamphetamine [20]. CYP2B6 metabolizes cocaine, phencyclidine, and some amphetamines. Both CYP2B6 and CYP2D6 are also induced by nicotine.

Pharmacodynamics

Pharmacodynamics is the study of the dose-response of a drug. This consists of the biochemical and physiological effects of the drugs on the body and how the body responds to maintain homeostasis. Drug dose may be plotted on a logarithmic scale which allows for mathematical manipulation of different dosages. The maximal effect of a drug is known as E_{max}. Efficacy is the extent of functional change imparted to a receptor. Efficacy is determined by the type of receptor and its effects on the body. Potency, however, is determined by the affinity of the receptor for the drug. It is the amount of drug needed to produce the given effect. Concentration of the drug needed to produce 50 % maximal effect occurs at EC_{50}. The more potent the drug, the smaller the dose required to achieve maximal effect.

Receptor binding may also be calculated with a log description noted that 50 % of a drug bound to receptors is K_d Maximum receptor binding is noted as B_{max}. Utilizing this information drug dosing may be calculated to understand the effects of the drug at different doses. This allows for the calculation in experiments of the median effective dose (ED_{50}), median toxic dose (TD_{50}), and median lethal dose (LD_{50}). The therapeutic index of a drug is calculated as the ratio of the (TD_{50}) to the (ED_{50}).

Receptors

Receptors contain two functional domains: ligand-binding sites and an effector or signaling area. Receptors are grouped according to four common types: ligand-gated ion channels, G protein-coupled receptor signaling, receptors with intrinsic enzymatic activity (guanylate cyclase, serine/threonine kinase, tyrosine kinase activity, tyrosine phosphatases), and receptors regulating nuclear transcription.

Ligand-gated ion channel receptors selectively gate the flow of ions through channels into the cell. Each one of these multisubunit proteins spans the plasma membrane several times forming a pore. Binding of these units enables them to control channel opening and closing. Excitatory neurotransmitters (acetylcholine and glutamate) result in a net inward current of cations like sodium, calcium, and potassium, which depolarizes the cell and increases generation of action potentials. Inhibitory neurotransmitters (GABA and glycine) result in net inward flux of anions like chloride which hyperpolarize the cell and decrease the generation of action potentials.

G proteins are coupled to what are commonly called serpentine receptors since they traverse the cell membrane an average of seven times. They posses an extracellular amino (N) terminal and an intracellular carboxyl (C) terminal. Drugs bind to the G protein receptors in the extracellular fluid and change the conformation of the receptor to activate the G protein. They may exist as dimmers or even large complexes. Dimerization may influence ligand preferences and/or regulate the affinity and specificity of the complex for G protein. Examples of G protein receptors include muscarinic acetylcholinergic receptors, receptors for adrenergic amines, serotonin receptors, and peptide hormone receptors. G proteins modify the activity of regulatory proteins and/or ion channels, which alter the activity of intracellular second messengers that enable the signal transduction and amplification. Cells of different tissues may have different G protein-dependent responses to the same initial ligand (norepinephrine, acetylcholine, serotonin).

Second messenger systems include the cyclic adenosine monophosphate (cAMP) (by means of G_s and G_1), cyclic guanosine monophosphate (cGMP), and phosphoinositides. Beta-adrenergic amines, glucagon, histamine, serotonin, and other hormones act on G_s to increase adenylyl cyclase and then increase the second messenger cAMP, while 2-adrenergic amines, muscarinic acetylcholine, opioids, serotonin, and others act on G_{i1}, G_{i2}, and G_{i3} to decrease adenylyl cyclase and then decrease cAMP. cAMP stimulates specific cAMP-dependent protein kinases that are differentially expressed in various tissues. When cAMP binds the regulatory dimer (D) of the kinase, two catalytic (C) chains are released which diffuse through the cytoplasm and nucleus, transferring phosphate from adenosine triphosphate(ATP) to other specific enzymes and substrate proteins.

G protein receptors may rapidly decrease their effects by reversible and rapid desensitization. When agonists induce conformational changes in the receptor, the receptor binds and activates a family of G protein-coupled receptor kinases (GRKs). The activated GRK then phosphorylates serine residues in the receptor's carboxy terminal tail, increasing the affinity for beta-arrestin, which in turn diminishes the receptor's to interact with G_s reducing the effects of adenylyl cyclase and the agonist response.

Desensitization may be homologous or heterologous. Homologous desensitization demonstrates feedback to the receptor molecule itself, and, heterologous desensitization extends to the action of all the receptors that share a common signaling pathway. Heterologous desensitization may affect one or more downstream proteins that participate in signaling from other receptors as well. Agonists may also induce endocytosis and membrane trafficking of receptors. Endocytosis may result in either the receptor recycling through the plasma membrane with continued cellular responsiveness or cause the receptor trafficking to lysosomes such that the causes down-regulation and decreased cellular response. Increased endocytosis and recycling of opiate receptors has been shown to have continued morphine analgesia with reduced tolerance and dependence [21].

Receptors with intrinsic enzyme activity consist of extracellular growth factor or hormone-binding domains connected to the cytoplasmic enzyme domain by a hydrophobic segment that crosses the plasma membrane's lipid bilayer. The cytoplasmic enzyme domain may be a tyrosine kinase, a serine/threonine kinase, or a guanylate cyclase that starts the signaling sequence. Drugs may target the agonist-binding sites or the enzymatic activity of the receptor.

Receptors that regulate nuclear transcription are soluble DNA-binding proteins that bypass the plasma membrane to reach their intracellular targets. Examples include: the steroid family of androgens, progesterone, glucocorticoid, and mineralocorticoid receptors, thyroid/retinoid family of receptors (thyroid, vitamin D, retinoic acid), and orphan receptor family. Since these actions require synthesis of new proteins, they have a relatively slow onset and action.

Mechanisms of Action

Drugs of abuse usually activate the mesolimbic system by interacting with ion channel receptors, binding to G_{io}-coupled receptors, or interfering with monoamine transporters [22]. Substances utilizing the first two mechanisms usually inhibit GABA inhibitory interneurons resulting in the net release of dopamine. Drugs that act indirectly or directly upon ion channel receptors can additionally increase dopamine in the nucleus accumbens and ventral tegmental areas (VTAs). Drugs that interfere with monoamine transporters block the reuptake or stimulate nonvesicular release of dopamine, causing an accumulation of dopamine in target structures. Nicotine, benzodiazepines, phencyclidine, and ketamine work through the ionotropic receptors. Nicotine activates the nicotinic acetylcholine receptor, and the benzodiazepines are modulators of $GABA_A$ receptors, potassium inwardly rectifying or G protein activated inwardly, rectifying potassium channels (Kir3/GIRK), glycine receptors, N-methyl-D-aspartate (NMDA) receptors, and 5-HT receptors. Alcohol also inhibits ENT1, the equilibrium producing nucleoside transporter for adenosine reuptake, resulting in adenosine accumulation, stimulation of adenosine A_2 receptors, and enhanced cAMP response to element-binding (CREB) protein signaling. Neither phencyclidine nor ketamine is physically addictive or associated with withdrawal but may lead to long-lasting psychosis due to noncompetitive antagonism of the NMDA receptor. With inhalants, nitric oxide acts on NMDA receptors while the fuel addictives enhance $GABA_A$ receptor function.

Opioids, cannabinoids, gamma-hydroxybutyric acid, and the hallucinogens all exert their action through G_{io}. The mu, kappa, and deltoid receptors all inhibit adenylyl cyclase but produce different neuronal effects. Mu opioid agonists inhibit GABA inhibition of dopamine with the net release of mesolimbic dopamine, reinforcement, and euphoria. However, kappa agonists inhibit dopamine neurons and induce dysphoria.

Cannabinoids cause presynaptic inhibition. The lipid-soluble neurotransmitters 2-arachidonoyl glycerol and anandamide bind to CB1 receptors to induce retrograde signaling from post- to presynaptic neurons where they may inhibit the release of either glutamate or GABA. Hallucinogens like LSD, mescaline, and psilocybin neither stimulate dopamine release nor cause addiction. These drugs act through $5\text{-}HT_{2A}$ receptor which couples to G_q proteins and inositol triphosphate (IP_3) and leads to intracellular calcium release. Hallucinogens by enhancing excitatory afferent input from the thalamus and increasing glutamate release in the cortex. Cocaine, amphetamine, methamphetamine, and ecstasy bind to transporters of biogenic amines. Cocaine inhibits the dopamine transporter, decreasing dopamine clearance from the synaptic cleft and causing an increase in extracellular dopamine. Amphetamine competitively inhibits dopamine transport at the dopamine transporter and interferes with the vesicular monoamine transporter to lessen the storage of dopamine in the synaptic vesicles. As cytoplasmic dopamine increases, there is reversal of the dopamine transporter, increasing the nonvesicular release of dopamine and further increasing extracellular dopamine. Ecstasy or MDMA is similar to amphetamine and causes release of biogenic amines by reversing the serotonin and other transporters.

G protein-coupled receptors may exist in multiple conformational states that include active, inactive, partially active, and selectively active. Drugs may bind at these sites as well. The affinity of the drug for the receptor will determine how much effect the drug has on the patient. Full agonists have a higher affinity for the active conformation and drive the equilibrium toward the active state. Partial agonists bind to the receptor with only moderate affinity for the active than for the inactive receptor. Even at saturation levels, partial agonists do no enable a full biologic response. An example is buprenorphine as a highly potent mu receptor agonist. It has a high affinity for the mu receptor and actually will displace morphine, methadone and other full opiate agonists from receptors. However, since it is not a full agonist, increases in dosages do not increase pharmacologic effects. Thus, higher doses of buprenorphine may be given without respiratory depression.

Antagonists have no effect upon response when used alone. They bind with equal affinity to the active and inactive conformations to prevent an agonist from inducing a response [23]. Inverse agonists have preferential affinity for inactive receptor conformations when otherwise the equilibrium would be shifted toward an active receptor. They, therefore, produce an effect opposite to those of an agonist. An example of this is a GABA-gated chloride ion channel agonist. This produces an inhibition of hyperpolarizing postsynaptic potentials. Their activity produce a range of sedative, anxiolytic, and anticonvulsant effects. The barbiturates and benzodiazepines both act at the GABA receptor. Benzodiazepines increase the frequency of the GABA-mediated chloride ion channel opening, and barbiturates increase the duration of the openings [24].

Tolerance and sensitization reflect changes in the way the body responds to a drug when it is used repeatedly. Tolerance is the reduction in response to a drug after its repeated administration. Tolerance shifts the dose-response curve to the right, requiring higher doses than the initial dose to achieve the same effect. Sensitization means that there is an increased drug response after its repeated administration. Repeated doses cause a greater effect after the initial dose. Some examples include cocaine which has its euphoria tolerance occur more rapidly than the cardiovascular effects. This may lead to massive overdoses of drugs to try an obtain the "rush" leading to toxic overdose effects.

Tolerance may occur by several mechanisms. Pharmacokinetic tolerance develops due to increased metabolism of a drug after repeated exposure with less of the drug being available in the bloodstream. For instance, microsomal ethanol-metabolizing enzymes, may be activated with prolonged ethanol exposure. Pharmacodynamic tolerance refers to the adaptive changes in receptor density, efficiency of receptor coupling, and/or signal transduction pathways that occur after repeated drug exposure. Learned tolerance refers to a reduction in the effects of a drug because of compensatory mechanisms that are learned. This may be seen in roofers and workers who are able to maintain their balance in the face of alcohol abuse. Conditioned tolerance is a subset of learned tolerance that occurs when a specific environment cues to drug administration. In fact, so powerful is the effect that the drug's action may be experienced before the drug is taken [25]. Cross-tolerance develops when the tolerance to repeated use of a specific drug in a given category is generalized to other drugs in same structural category. The cross-tolerance that occurs between alcohol, barbiturates, and benzodiazepines may be used to provide weaning of a patient during drug detoxification. Physical dependence is a state that develops as a result of the adaptation produced by the resetting homeostatic mechanisms after repeated drug use. Physical dependence can arise from many sources, addictive and nonaddictive.

Alcohol

Alcohol is the chemical name for a group of related compounds that contains a hydroxyl group (–OH) bound to a carbon atom. The form consumed by humans is ethyl alcohol or ethanol consisting of two carbons and a single hydroxyl group (written as C_2H_2OH or C_6H_6O). This class of substances includes beer, wines, and distilled spirits. A standard alcohol drink is defined as one that contains 0.6 fluid ounces of alcohol. This is the amount of alcohol in a 12 oz can of beer, 5 oz of wine, or 1.5 oz of distilled spirits (40 % ethanol by volume). Alcohol is a small, water-soluble molecule is rapidly and efficiently absorbed into the bloodstream from the stomach, small intestine, and colon. Rate of absorption depends on the gastric emptying time and can be delayed by the presence of food in the small intestine. Once in the bloodstream, alcohol is rapidly distributed throughout the body and gains access to all tissues, including the fetus in the pregnant.

The relationship between alcohol intake and blood levels is weight dependent. Gender is important with women showing a 20–25 % higher blood alcohol level than men with the same amount of alcohol ingested. Most of alcohol is metabolized by enzymes with a small amount excreted through the lungs as vapor. In the liver, alcohol is broken down by ADH and mixed function oxidases of P4500IIE1 (CYP2E1). Levels of CYP2E1 may be increased in chronic drinkers. ADH converts alcohol to acetaldehyde, which may be converted to acetate by the actions of acetaldehyde dehydrogenase. The rate of alcohol metabolism by ADH is relatively constant, as the enzyme is saturated at low blood alcohol levels and exhibits zero-order kinetics (constant amount oxidized per unit of time). Alcohol metabolism is proportional to body weight (and liver weight) and averages approximately 1 oz of pure alcohol per 3 h in adults. There are no effective "alcohol antagonists" that will reverse intoxicating effects of alcohol. Naloxone, the opiate antagonist, has been tested for its ability to reverse alcohol-induced coma but appears ineffective [26]. Several gamma-aminobutyric acid$_A$ (GABA$_A$) receptor antagonists have also been evaluated including flumazenil (Anexate) and metadoxine (pyridoxal L-2-pyrrolidone-5-carboxylate) appears to increase clearance of alcohol and speed recovery [27].

Alcohol acts acutely as a central nervous system (CNS) depressant. During the initial phase when blood alcohol levels are rising, a period of disinhibition often occurs and signs of behavioral arousal are common. These include relief of anxiety, increased talkativeness, feelings of confidence and euphoria, and enhanced assertiveness. As the drinking continues, there are impairments in judgment and reaction time, increased emotional outbursts, and ataxia. At higher blood levels, alcohol acts as a sedative and hypnotic, although the quality of sleep may be reduced after alcohol intake. In patients with sleep apnea, alcohol increases the severity and frequency of episodes. It may also potentiate the sedative–hypnotic properties of benzodiazepines and barbiturates. Alcohol also enhances the sedative effects of antihistamines and the liver toxic effects of acetaminophen and the gastric irritation effects of NSAIDs increasing the risk of gastritis and upper GI bleeding.

Alcohol effects the reward pathway by enhancing the release of dopamine from the midbrain dopaminergic projections that regulate neurotransmission within the limbic and cortical circuits that regulate motivated behavior [28]. The dopamine (DA) neurons involved in this action reside in the midbrain VTA and project to discrete areas of the brain, including the nucleus accumbens, olfactory tubercle, frontal cortex, amygdale, and septal/Hippocampal areas. These regions are thought to be involved in translating emotion and perception into action through the activation of motor pathways; thus, they may be important in initiating and sustaining drug-seeking behavior. Lesions or inactivation of these discrete brain areas in animals can reduce both the acquisition of drug seeking and its reinstatement following long periods of abstinence.

The initial reinforcing action of alcohol appears to involve the excitation of VTA dopamine neurons. Initially, alcohol enhances the firing rate of the midbrain DA neurons. Chronic exposure to alcohol leads to alternations in the excitability of these neurons in the absence of alcohol that may persist for significant periods of time. Electrophysiologic studies have demonstrated enhanced efficiency of glutamatergic signaling in neurons following exposure to alcohol and other drugs of abuse [29–31]. Human studies with selective pharmacologic agents found neurotransmitters like GABA, serotonin, and opiates mediate the rewarding and craving of alcohol addiction. Imaging studies are now being done to identify changes in brain activation during exposure to alcohol or alcohol-related cues between control and alcohol-dependent subjects [32, 33].

Psychostimulants like cocaine, amphetamines, or opiates like heroin and morphine all produce their primary effects by binding to specific protein receptors expressed on brain neurons. By contrast, alcohol interacts with a wide variety of targets including both lipids and proteins. Alcohol's acute depressant action on neuronal excitability results from its influence on the function of inhibitory ion channels while it blocks the activity of excitatory receptors.

Alcohol usually potentiates $GABA_A$ and glycine receptor function. However, the subset of $GABA_A$-rho receptors are inhibited by alcohol. Both the gamma-$GABA_A$ and delta-GABA receptors are acutely sensitive to low levels of alcohol. Both of these GABA receptors contain the alpha-4, beta, and delta subunit receptors instead of the gamma receptors and appear to be affected by only 5–10 mM of alcohol consistent with only a single drink [34]. Further evidence has also been found to demonstrate the effects of alcohol's effects on the presynaptic release of GABA instead of the GABA receptors. The amygdala appears to show affects on the release of GABA from the postsynaptic regions rather than the GABA receptors [35].

The major excitatory neurotransmitter is glutamate which has three major subtypes of ion channels that activate the brain. These ion channels are AMPA, kainate, and NMDA receptors. AMPA is alpha-amino-3 hydroxy-5-methyl-4-isoxazolepropionic acid. The ion channels control the majority of the fast excitatory synaptic transmissions in the brain and critical mediators of most of the types of synaptic plasticity involved in learning and memory. NMDA receptors need both glutamate and glycine for activation and are extremely calcium permeable. The AMPA and kainate receptors, however, only need glutamate to function. NMDA receptors are inhibited by alcohol, nitrous oxide, anesthetics, and volatile solvents like toluene [36]. NMDA receptors have sensitivity to varying concentrations of alcohol. AMPA and kainate receptors have a more selective ethanol receptor sensitivity. The NMDA receptors are antagonized by alcohol concentrations at 10–100 mM and are associated with intoxication and sedation. NMDA demonstrates regional differences most likely due to differential expression of GluN1 and GluN2 NMDA subunits [37, 38]. The blocking of excitatory NMDA signals appears to be critical the intoxicating and sedative effects of effects of alcohol. Inhibition of NMDA receptors in the prefrontal cortex likely contributes to the cognitive and judgment errors with alcohol intoxication [39]. Long-term alcohol use may also affect NMDA receptors in the medial and orbital cortical areas which are necessary for adapting behavior to changing environment. The NMDA receptors are also important in the regulation of dopamine release in the mesolimbic region of the nucleus accumbens.

The 5-HT$_3$ receptors are ligand-gated ion channels activated by serotonin. Studies show that 5-HT$_3$ receptor antagonists block the ability to discriminate alcohol from saline which may explain the subjective effects of alcohol.

Acetylcholine activates a group of ligand-gated ion channels expressed in brain neurons that are similar to the nicotinic receptors found at the neuromuscular junctions [40]. Alcohol appears to have both inhibitory and excitatory effects on acetylcholine receptors. These effects seem to be related to the various subunits of nicotine. The alpha-beta subunits appear potentiated by ethanol and the alpha subunits (alpha-7) are inhibited by ethanol. It is known that nicotinic receptors are expressed by neurons in the VTA, nucleus accumbens, and prefrontal cortex where they assist in the excitability of the neurons.

ATP-gated ion channels release ATP into the synapses where it exerts its influence on the ATP-gated channels of the 2PX family [41]. The actions on the P2X receptors is subtype specific. The PX2 and P2X4 receptors are inhibited by alcohol and the PsX3 receptors are facilitated.

Potassium and calcium-selective ion channels regulated by calcium and those by G proteins (SK and BK channels) are directly and indirectly affected by alcohol. Potassium channels inhibit excitatory glutamatergic transmissions by hyperpolarizing the membrane. BK channel activity is activated by alcohol and this is thought to inhibit the release of vasopressin from the neurohypophysial terminal and result in diuresis. SK channels do not appear to be inhibited by ethanol but their expression and localization in Hippocampal neurons are changed by chronic alcohol usage. This may be part of the cause of the ethanol withdrawal excitability. Alterations in T-type calcium channels in thalamic neurons caused by alcohol use may cause sleep problems seen in ethanol-dependent individuals.

Adenosine functions as a significant inhibitory neurotransmitter in the brain and as a possible endogenous antiepileptic due to its ability to inhibit neuronal function. Alcohol inhibits the function of nucleoside transporters leading to increased intracellular adenosine levels.

Increases in the activity of the mesolimbic projecting dopamine neurons are important in reinforcing the effects of alcohol abuse. Alcohol increases the firing of dopamine neurons that a found in the VTA causing increased dopamine release in the nucleus accumbens [42].

Endogenous opioids (endorphins and enkephalins) along with other neuropeptides have been linked to ethanol addiction. Alcohol increases blood levels of beta-endorphins in humans [43].

Endocannabinoids (EC) appear to be a significant actor in alcohol use [44]. ECs are lipid-derived molecules that activate receptors (CB1, CB2) and also bind THC the psychoactive part of marijuana. ECs regulate the GABAergic and glutamatergic synaptic transmission and are synthesized during periods of significant neuronal depolarization.

Nonalcohol Sedative Hypnotics

Sedative–hypnotic drugs are a diverse group of drugs that suppress CNS activity. They are most commonly used as anxiolytics, hypnotics, anticonvulsants, muscle relaxants, and anesthesia inducing agents. This includes benzodiazepines, nonbenzodiazepines hypnotics, barbiturates, and other compounds. The basic structure of the benzodiazepines is the 1,4-benzodiazepine nucleus. Alterations of the structure change the efficacy, potency, and other properties of the different drugs. Substitutions on the benzodiazepine ring structure have produced: (a) the triazole group: alprazolam, triazolam, and estazolam; (b) 2-keto group: diazepam, flurazepam, and clorazepate; (c) the 2-amino-group: chlordiazepoxide; (d) the 3-hydroxy group: lorazepam, oxazepam, and temazepam; (e) the trifluoroethyl group: quazepam; (f) the imidazole group: midazolam; and (g) the 7-nitrogroup: nitrazepam and clonazepam. There are four other nonbenzodiazepine hypnotics that also have hypnotic effects due to the gamma-aminobutyric acid ($GABA_A$) receptors. These include: (a) zopiclone, a cyclopyrrolone; (b) eszopiclone, a stereoselective isomer zopiclone; (c) zaleplon, a pyrazolopyrimidine; and (d) zolpidem, an imidazopyridine [45–47]. All these drugs operate at the gamma-butyric acid receptors but not exactly like benzodiazepines.

Benzodiazepines including alprazolam, lorazepam, and diazepam are very common psychiatric medications. Most benzodiazepines have hepatic metabolism involving oxidative reactions mediated by the cytochrome P450 (CYP450) enzymes. Oxidative metabolism involves N-dealkylation or aliphatic hydroxylation. The VYP3A4 enzyme controls the oxidative metabolism of many of the benzodiazepines and is active in the biotransformation of the nonbenzodiazepine sedative–hypnotics: eszopiclone, zaleplon, and zolpidem. A number of the benzodiazepines are converted into active metabolites like desmethyldiazepam that have long half-lives. The final common pathway usually involves conjugation of the parent drug or the metabolites with glucuronide. The drugs or metabolites that undergo glucuronidation have a hydroxyl group attached. Those with parent drugs, like lorazepam and oxazepam, with direct glucuronidation have less drug interaction and reduced clearance with impaired liver function when compared to other benzodiazepines.

The other nonbenzodiazepine hypnotics appear to have unique metabolic pathways for their metabolism. Zolpidem is metabolized by CYP3A4, CYP2C9, and CYP29 into inactive metabolites by hydroxylation [48]. Aldehyde dehydrogenase appears to have a major part in the metabolism of zaleplon. Zaleplon converts to the metabolite of 5-oxozaleplon with urinary excretion. Zopiclone converts to a decarboxylated metabolite via an esterase and is excreted through the lungs. It is also converted by CYP3A4 into an active metabolite zopi-

clone N-oxide and an inactive metabolite of
N-desmethylzopiclone.

Benzodiazepines and abuse appears complex. The quick
onset of action appears to produce euphoria. The onset of
action after oral administration is influenced by the formulation of the drug, the intrinsic activity, lipid solubility, protein
binding, and rate of entry into the brain. It is thought that
greater lipid solubility enhances uptake in the brain with
diazepam more rapidly entering the brain than lorazepam.
However, the pharmacokinetics may not predict abuse. Certain
medications, such as clonazepam, are rapidly absorbed and
quickly reach high plasma levels, yet do not produce the
euphoria sought by abusing individuals when compared to
lorazepam. Lower abuse potential follows the need to convert prodrugs into active metabolites in the liver. An example
is formation of desmeythldiazepam from halazepam which is
much less likely to be abused compared to diazepam.

The benzodiazepines and the benzodiazepine receptor
agonists exert their effects via the allosteric modulation of
the $GABA_A$ receptors. The inhibitory effects of the GABA
receptors by the benzodiazepines is the reason these medications are sedative, anticonvulsants, hypnotic, and amnesia
producing. $GABA_A$ receptors are a hetropentameric protein
scaffolding surrounded by a central chloride channel [49].
The receptors may be activated by direct agonists like musci-
mol, which leads to an influx of chloride ions, or, indirectly by
drugs such as the benzodiazepines which enhance GABA
binding to the receptor with increased frequency of opening
the chloride channel. There are five subunits have several
subtypes (alpha, beta, gamma, delta, epsilon, rho, and pi)
which each have a specific amino acid sequence. There are
also multiple subtypes in each category that inhabit various
regions of the brain. Benzodiazepines bind primarily the
gamma-2 and alpha subunits. Alpha-1 subunits are found in
the frontal, cortex, and other cortical areas, globus pallidus,
hippocampus substantia nigra, and cerebellum. $GABA_A$
of the alpha-5 subunit are seen in the limbic regions [50].
Receptors with the alpha-1, alpha-2, alpha-3, and alpha-5

subunits all react to the benzodiazepines. The alpha-5 receptor operates extrasynaptically and regulates the tonic GABAergic currents while the other three are found in the synapse and modulate the GABA rapid-phase currents. The alpha-4 and alpha-6 receptors cause a lack of sensitivity to the benzodiazepines.

The alpha-1 receptors control the sedative–hypnotic effects of the benzodiazepines [51]. There is also evidence to support this subunit may be the source of the ataxia with benzodiazepines and zolpidem. Antianxiety receptors include the alpha-2 and alpha-3 subunits [52]. The alpha-2 and alpha-3 subunits may also be involved in the muscle relaxation and reward aspects of benzodiazepines.

Barbiturates possess pharmacodynamic properties of the benzodiazepines. At lower concentrations, the barbiturates modulate $GABA_A$ receptors with allosteric modification. At the higher concentrations, barbiturates are direct $GABA_A$ agonists that open the chloride channels. Barbiturates appear to reduce excitatory neurotransmission by inhibition of alpha-amino-3-hydroxy-5-methyl-4-isoxazolepropionic acid (AMPA) receptors and also inhibit neurotransmitter release by blocking voltage-sensitive calcium channels. The nonbarbiturate hypnotics as positive modulators of the effects of GABA agonists on $GABA_A$ receptors. They act very similarly to the benzodiazepines producing sedative–hypnotic, anxiolytic, myorelaxation, and anticonvulsant effects. They appear to have less amnestic effects and less tolerance. Differences in the binding affinities for different $GABA_A$ receptor subtypes are reflected in the potency of the positive $GABA_A$ receptor modulators to enhance the GABA-mediated currents.

Serious drug interaction occurs with the use of sedative–hypnotics and alcohol. Benzodiazepines that are metabolized through the CYP3A4 pathway may have adverse effects by other drugs. Some inhibitors include ketoconazole, itraconazole, macrolide antibiotics (EES), fluoxetine, nefazodone, and cimetidine. Combined contraceptives may alter the metabolism of substrates of CYP1A2, CYP3A4, and CYP2C19.

Inducers of P450, such as rifampin, may increased clearance of the nonbarbiturate hypnotics with decreased plasma levels. Barbiturates in particular are extremely dangerous when take with alcohol or used in high doses due to CNS depression. Barbiturates may induce their own metabolism with reduced therapeutic effects (CYP2B6, CYP2C9, CYP3A4).

The sedative–hypnotics have three characteristics in the production of addiction: hedonic effects, tolerance, and withdrawal syndrome. Hedonistic effects with the benzodiazepines not commons since they do not produce euphoria unless used with other drugs. Tolerance is most commonly seen when the medications are used as hypnotics but less commonly for anxiety. The withdrawal from benzodiazepines may be significant and even seizures may occur. The $GABA_A$ receptors appear to decrease in responsiveness in the development of tolerance. There may also be alteration in the receptor subtypes with chronic exposure that alters responsiveness. The glutamatergic system may also have a major role in the benzodiazepine withdrawal by the upregulation of Hippocampal AMPA receptors and the conductance of APMA-controlled neurons.

Benzodiazepines have definite abuse potential and those with the most likelihood are flunitrazepam, diazepam, alprazolam, and lorazepam. The lowest likelihood are clonazepam, chlordiazepoxide, halazepam, prazepam, quazepam, and oxazepam. Much of this is related to rapidity of onset with a feeling of well-being, relief of anxiety, and relaxation.

Opioids

There are three types of opioid receptors found in the nervous system: mu, kappa, and delta. The usual opioid analgesics act mostly as agonists or partial agonists at mu receptors. Heroin and most of the compounds derived from opium and man-made analogs act at the opioid receptors as agonists. The three natural endogenous opioids also act as agonists: beta-endorphins, enkephalins, and dynorphins. There is some selectivity for the receptor classes The beta-endorphins have a high affinity fro mu and delta receptors with lower affinity for kappa receptors. The dynorphins, however, have a selectivity for kappa receptors over the mu and delta receptors. The mu receptor appears to be the most clinically relevant of the three. Beta-endorphin is produced in the anterior pituitary from proopiomelanocortin. It is further produced in the CNS and the periphery. The mu receptors control both the analgesic and pleasurable effects of opioid compounds. The also modulate effects in the hypothalamic-pituitary-adrenal (HPA) axis, immune, gastrointestinal, and pulmonary regions.

The opioids include all the compounds, natural, and synthetic that are related to opium poppies and endogenous opioid neuropeptides.

Heroin is a synthetically manufactured natural opioid alkaloid morphine. Due to the rapidity of onset and short half-life, heroin is a classic and popular drug for abuse. It is a Schedule I drug with no therapeutic use. Heroin is a prodrug that is not active itself. Heroin is rapidly deacetylated to 6-monoacetyl morphine and morphine which are active at the mu receptors. Heroin is a prodrug that is more water soluble and potent than morphine. It is synthesized from morphine by acetylation at the 3 and 6 positions and metabolized in humans to active opioid compounds initially by deacetylation to the 6-monoacetylmorphine (6-MAM), and then by further deacetylation to morphine. Heroin has an average ½ life in humans of about 3 min and IV administration; the half-life of the metabolite 6-acetylmorphine is about 30 min in humans. Any use of heroin by the intranasal, IM, or IV routes produce peak blood levels within about 5 min but intranasal has about half the relative potency of IV or IM routes.

Morphine is a natural product of the opium poppy *Papaver somniferum*. Morphine is an alkaloid compound that belongs to the class of drugs called the phenanthrenes. This also includes codeine and thebaine. Synthetic modifications of the chemical structure of morphine at the 3, 6, and 17 positions produce other synthetic compounds including morphine-6-glucuronide (M6G). Related drugs include hydrocodone (Vicodin), oxycodone (OxyContin), hydromorphone (Dilaudid), and heroin. Synthetic compounds also include antagonists like naloxone (Narcan), naltrexone (Trexan), nalmefene (Revix) along with partial agonists like buprenorphine (subutex) and naloxone/ buprenorphine (suboxone) [53]. Morphine is mostly selective for MOP-r receptors and is biotransformed mostly by hepatic glucuronidation to the major inactive metabolite morphine-3-glucuronide (M3G) and the biologic M6G compound [55]. The pharmacokinetics or morphine and metabolites vary depending on the route of administration. Its oral bioavailability varies from 35 to 75 % with the plasma half-life of 2–3.5 h with the analgesic effect half-life of 4–6 h which reduces accumulation. It mostly cleared in the liver with the enterohepatic cycling with oral administration. Adjustment for renal disease is needed due to the clearance by the kidneys.

Oxycodone is used usually for moderate pain and popular for abuse when crushed and taken intranasally or IV. It is a semisynthetic compound derived from thebaine with agonist activity mostly at the mu receptors. It is pharmacologically similar to morphine as has a 1:2 equivalency to morphine. Onset of action begins 1 h after oral administration with the sustained release lasting for about 12 h and a plasma half-life for the immediate release of 3–4 h. Plasma levels stabilize within 24 h with oral bioavailability from 60 to 87 % with 45 % protein bound. Oxycodone is chiefly metabolized in the liver with the remainder processed in the kidneys. The two major metabolites are oxymorphone which is also a potent analgesic and noroxycodone which is weaker. Protein binding and lipophilicity is similar to morphine with a longer half-life and greater bioavailability. It is metabolized mostly by the cytochrome CYP2D6 enzyme.

Codeine is methyl morphine, with a methyl substitution on the phenolic hydroxyl group of morphine. It is more lipophilic than morphine and crosses the blood–brain barrier more rapidly. Also, has a large first-pass phenomenon in the liver with greater bioavailability then morphine but is less potent.

A small portion is metabolized to morphine by the cytochrome 2D6 system [53]. Codeine has a high oral-parental effect due to its low first-pass metabolism in the liver. Its metabolites are mostly inactive and excreted in the urine with 10 % demethylated by the CYP2D6 enzyme pathway to morphine. Morphine is responsible for the analgesic effects since codeine has a low activity for the opioid receptors. Genetic variations in the enzyme systems may cause a lower production of M6G with accumulation of the active metabolites in patients with poor renal clearance.

Meperidine is phenylpiperidine and has several forms. It is rarely used longer than 48 h or doses greater than 600 mg/day due to its toxicity. It is active in CNS and bowel. If used with MAOIs, it may produce a serotonergic effect with clonus, hyperreflexia, hyperthermia, and agitation. Onset of the analgesic effects begin after oral ingestion in about 15 min with the peak in 1–2 h with a duration of 1½–3 h [53]. The medication is absorbed by all routes but less reliable by IM routes. It is mostly metabolized in the liver with a half-life of about 3 h. Liver disease leads to increased half-life and bioavailability of meperidine and normeperidine. Sixty percent of the drug is excreted protein bound.

Pentazocine is available in oral and parenteral formulas. It is one of the first agonist–antagonist medications. It is a weak antagonist or partial agonist with a plateau effect at the mu and kappa receptors. Peak effect is ½–1 h with given orally and its duration of action is 3–6 h. Sixty percent is protein bound, and it is metabolized by the liver in the oxidative and glucuronide conjugation with a large first-pass effect. Oral bioavailability is about 10 % except with cirrhosis it may increase to 60–70 %. Half-life is about 2–3 h with small amounts excreted unchanged in the urine.

Hydromorphone is a potent opioid analgesic than morphine and is used for moderate to severe pain. It is excreted by the kidneys. It is available by IV, oral, and rectal routes. It is five times more potent per milligram than morphine orally and 8.5 times more potent when given IV. It is shorter acting than morphine. It has an oral bioavailability of

30–40 % with an analgesic onset after 10–20 min with a peak in 30–60 min with effects lasting for 3–5 h. The oral parenteral ratio is 5:1 with an equivalency of 1.5 mg of hydrocodone to 10 mg of morphine.

Hydrocodone is a mild pain reliever and often combined with acetaminophen. Hydrocodone has a half-life of 2–4 h with a peak efficacy at ½–1 h. Its duration of action is 3–4 h. It may show up in urine drug testing with codeine use since about 11 % of codeine is metabolized to hydrocodone therefore giving a false-positive testing.

Methadone is a synthetic long-acting full mu opioid agonist active by oral and parenteral routes. Its primary use is in heroin addiction as a substitute medication. The $l^®$-methadone enantiomer has up to 50 times more analgesic activity and the potential for respiratory depression than the d(S)-enantiomer. Both forms have modest NMDA receptor antagonism. Methadone has a diphenylheptylamine structure and is a racemic mix of both d(S)- and l(R)-methadone. Both the enantiomers are weak NMDA receptor antagonists and therefore retards and attenuates the development of opioid tolerance. It meets the two most important criteria for use with addictions: high systemic bioavailability (>90 %) with oral administration and long half-life with long-term administration. Oral methadone is rapidly absorbed bur has delayed onset of action with peak plasma levels at 2–4 h and sustained over a 24 h time frame. Further, the mean terminal half-life of racemic d,l-methadone is about 24 h and the l-enantiomer with a half-life of 36 h. Chronic administration accumulates methadone in the liver and levels remain constant due to the slow release of unmetabolized drug into the bloodstream with more than 90 % plasma protein bound. Due to the long half-life, the medication must be increased slowly by 10 mg every 4–7 days (initial dosing 20–40 mg/day). Some patients are rapid metabolizers with increased clearance by the P450-enzyme or p-glycoprotein-related transporter systems. Levels of methadone generally peak at 3–8 h after administration. Methadone is biotransformed in the liver by the cytochrome P450-related enzymes (CYP3A4 in the majority and to a lesser extent the CYP2B6, CYP2D6, and CYP1A2 systems) [56]. It is biotransformed into the two N-demethylated biologically inactive metabolites that then undergo further oxidative metabolism. It is excreted in almost equal amounts in the urine and feces. It patients with renal disease, the drug may be cleared entirely by the GI route. Severe liver disease may cause decreased methadone levels due to decreased storage. Use of medications that alter the cytochrome P450 enzyme system must be used with caution. This includes rifampin, rifabutin, carbamazepine, phenytoin, and phenobarbital. Also, consumption of more than four drinks in a day have been shown to alter methadone levels.

Levo-alpha-acetylmethadol (LAAM) is a synthetic, longer acting form (48 h) of methadone that is orally effective. LAAM has had problems with prolonged QT interval and *torsade de pointes* and is no longer available in the USA.

Buprenorphine alone and combined with naloxone was approved in 2002 by the FDA as a sublingual treatment for heroin and opioid addiction and rescheduled to a Schedule III medication. Buprenorphine is an MOP-r-directed partial agonist and also a partial kappa agonist. It structurally a oripavine with a C7 side chain with a tert-butyl group. Norbuprenorphine is the major metabolite with activity at the MOP-r receptors as well. Buprenorphine is metabolized to norbuprenorphine due to dealkylation in the cytochrome P450-related enzyme 3A4 system which buprenorphine is a weak inhibitor [57]. The drug undergoes rapid first pass in the liver with sublingual bioavailability of 50–60 %. There have been several deaths reported with buprenorphine and benzodiazepines. It also has some weak kappa opioid receptor activity. Due to ceiling effects of the drug, doses greater than 32 mg sublingually do not have any further effects on the mu MOP-r receptors. It has a long half-life of 24–48 h because of its slow dissociation from the MOP-r receptors. IV dosing has a plasma half-life of 3–5 h. Oral administration is not very effective due to its first-pass phenomenon.

Opioids generally are abused as agonists of the MOP-receptors (mu-encoded receptors at OPRM1 receptor gene) [54]. MOP-r are G protein-coupled 7-transmembrane domain receptors. They are coupled to G_i and G_o proteins and result in acute downstream decrease in adenylate cyclase activity. The MOP-r receptors are widely found in the CNS, and their effects are mediated in different areas of the CNS. Therapeutic analgesic effects are found in the dorsal spinal column and thalamus while respiratory depression is found in the brainstem. The receptors are also active in the locus ceruleus and other centers to produce physiologic dependence and withdrawal. The abuse and addiction effects are thought to be found in the ventral and dorsal striatal areas with effects on the dopaminergic mesocorticolimbic and nigrostriatal systems.

Cocaine, Amphetamines, stimulants

Stimulants include the naturally occurring plant alkaloids including cocaine, ephedra, and khat as well as the synthetic compounds like amphetamines and methylphenidate. Most of these stimulants are modifications of the basic phenethylamine structure which is similar to endogenous catecholamine neurotransmitters norepinephrine and dopamine. The stimulant all have similar psychological and physiologic characteristics.

Cocaine

Cocaine is an alkaloid with a tropane ester structure similar to scopolamine and other plant alkaloids. The compound is found in the leaves of the *Erythoxylum coca*. The leaves contain approximately 0.2–1 % cocaine and several other tropane alkaloids of unknown activity. Cocaine has two stereoisomers: (−)-cocaine and (+)-cocaine which has less affinity for the dopamine transporter and is relatively inactive due to rapid metabolism by butyrylcholinesterase.

Ephedra

Ephedrine and pseudoephedrine are naturally occurring alkaloids with phenethylamine chemical structure and are found in several of the *Ephedraceae* plant species. It is prepared from the dried young branches of the plants. It then is taken as a capsule, tincture, liquid extract, or tea. Synthetic ephedrine and pseudoephedrine are also available for consumption. The ephedra alkaloids have the same range of psychological and physiological effects that cocaine and amphetamines do. These compounds have been linked to severe cardiovascular and CNS problems and, thus, their ban in the USA in 2006.

Khat

This is the common name for any preparations of the *Catha edulis* plant native to East Africa and in the southern Arabian peninsula. Fresh khat leaves contain two stimulant alkaloids with phenethylamine chemical structure: cathinone (1–3 %) and cathine (norpseudoephedrine). Pure cathinone is a Schedule I substance and cathine is a Schedule IV substance. Cathinone has action and potency similar to amphetamines [58]. Potent synthetic cathinones include mephedrone, methylone, and 3,4-methylenedioxypyrovalerone which are sold as "bath salts."

Synthetic Stimulants

There are over a dozen synthetic stimulant medications legally available in the USA by either prescription or over the counter. Most of the medications are variations from the basic phenethylamine structure. All legal stimulants are sold as tablets, capsules, or in the liquid form. The extend release formulations are used for the treatment of attention deficit disorder (ADD). Also methylphenidate may be used a transdermal patch. Amphetamine is available as a prodrug lisdexamfetamine which is a *d*-amphetamine with the amino acid L-lysine. Active drug is formed when the lysine is hydrolyzed off in the intestines and liver. This allows for longer duration of action and reduced abuse potential. Some OTC medications have aerosolized forms for use as decongestants. Amphetamines are usually abused by the oral or IV route. Also, the pure crystallized methamphetamine may be used intranasally, or smoked, like cocaine. Illicit "meth labs" make methamphetamine by reducing ephedrine or pseudoephedrine. Stimulants with the phenylisopropylamine structure (amphetamine, methamphetamine, ephedrine, pseudoephedrine, and phenylpropanolamine) have a chiral, or stereoisomeric, center a the alpha-carbon atom and exist in two or more stereoisomeric forms that have differing pharmacodynamic and pharmacokinetic properties. The *d*- or *S*-(+) isomer has 3–5 times the CNSA activity and about 1/3 the half-life of the *l*- or *R* (−) isomer. The *l*-isomers have more peripheral alpha-adrenergic activity. For instance, *d*-methamphetamine is a strong CNS stimulant while *l*-methamphetamine has uses as a decongestant (as in a nasal inhaler). Methylphenidate has four stereoisomers with the *d*-threo as the active drug.

Pharmacokinetics

Route of administration greatly effects the pharmacokinetics of the stimulants. Smoked stimulants (cocaine/amphetamine) are quickly absorbed and reach the brain in 6–8 s. The onset and peak are within minutes of administration. The redistribution of the stimulant from the brain leads to a rapid decline in effects. IV administration has peak brain uptake in 4–7 min based on the positron emission tomography (PET) scans with radiolabeled cocaine [59]. The highest levels of cocaine are found in the striatum (Caudate, putamen, and nucleus accumbens) and the lowest in the orbital cortex and cerebellum. Clearance to the half-peak levels in the brain takes 17–30 min and is most rapidly cleared from the orbital cortex, thalamus, and cerebellum with slowest clearing in the striatum. The rapid decline in the levels is described as a "crash" by users. Intranasal and oral stimulants have a slower absorption and slower onset of effect (30–45 min), a longer peak effect, and a more gradual decline from peak levels. The peak intensity with oral use relates to the peak cocaine plasma concentration which is generally about half that of intranasal cocaine. Cocaine is well absorbed in mucous membranes, intact skin, or even passive inhalation of aerosolized particles of smoked cocaine. Stimulants may enter most tissues. Cocaine rapidly distributes to the heart, kidney, adrenal glands, and liver. In concert with blood and urine, cocaine and its hydrolytic metabolites, amphetamines, phentermine, and ephedrine and its analogs may be found in hair, sweat, saliva, nails, and breast milk. They also cross the placenta and are found in the umbilical cord blood, amniotic fluid, and meconium.

Metabolism of cocaine is 95 % by hydrolysis of ester bonds to benzoylecgonine (primary urinary metabolite) and ecgonine methyl ester by the action of the carboxylesterases in the liver and butyrylcholinesterase in the liver, plasma, brain, lung, and other tissues [60–62]. The remaining 5 % of cocaine is N-demethylated to norcocaine by the CYP3A4 isozyme of the liver cytochrome P450 microsomal enzyme system. Norcocaine has similar action to cocaine and is hepatotoxic. Amphetamines are metabolized in three separate pathways: deamination to inactive metabolite, oxidation to norephedrine and other active metabolites, and parahydroxylation to active metabolites. Most stimulants and their metabolites are eliminated in the urine. Benzoylecgonine is the highest level metabolite found in the urine and may be present for several days after last use.

Mechanism of Action of Stimulants

All stimulants act to enhance the extracellular concentration of the monoamine neurotransmitters (dopamine, norepinephrine, and serotonin) in the central and peripheral nervous system.

Stimulants act by disrupting the function of the plasma membrane transport system. Usually, the monoamine transporters control the uptake or reuptake of the previously released neurotransmitters from the extracellular space back into the nerve cells. These transporters are found not just at synapses but also on cell bodies, dendrites, and axons. Stimulant drugs fall into two classes based on their molecular mechanism of action: transporter blockers and transporter substrates. Transporter blockers include cocaine and methylphenidate that bind to the extracellular face of transporters and inhibit the uptake of previously released monoamine neurotransmitters. Transport blockers are often called uptake or reuptake blockers. Transporter substrates include amphetamine and phentermine. These drugs bind to transporters, move into the cell neuronal cytoplasm with sodium ions, and trigger the release of monoamines by reversing the normal direction of transporter flux. Inside the neuronal cytoplasm the transporters interact with vesicular monoamine transporters (VMAT) to move monoamines into the cytoplasm increasing the concentration available for release. Thus, these drugs are styled as releasers.

The potent stimulants such as cocaine and amphetamine act at the dopamine and norepinephrine transporters. Weaker stimulants such as (−)-ephedrine and its isomers target norepinephrine transporters. Stimulant drugs may also have other ancillary actions. Cocaine blocks the sodium channels and amphetamine inhibits monoamine oxidase.

Stimulants act centrally by activating the mesocorticolimbic dopamine system [63]. The pathway is thought to involve the cell bodies in the VTA that send axonal projections to the prefrontal cortex, nucleus accumbens, and amygdala. The mesocorticolimbic dopamine neurons are included in the cortical-striatal-pallidal system that is responsible for adaptive behavioral responses. The nucleus accumbens is the center critical to the circuitry receiving stimulatory glutamate afferents from the hippocampus, amygdala, and frontal cortex. The primary cell is the GABA-containing spiny neuron that has direct synaptic contact from the dopamine and glutamate neurons.

The spiny neurons send efferent projections to several target areas including pallidal structures in the substantia nigra pars reticulata that modulates tonic suppression of motor nuclei. Activation of the GABAergic spiny neurons recruit motor behaviors by inhibiting the pallidal output (via disinhibition). The spiny neurons include two types based upon their affinity for dopamine receptors: low-affinity D_1 dopamine receptors and high-affinity dopamine D_2 receptors. The spiny neurons respond to glutamate and the dopamine receptors differentially modulate the response to the glutamate. In general, the D_1 dopamine receptors increase the excitability of the spiny neurons and the D_2 receptors inhibit the spiny neurons. Thus, behaviors are either executed (D_1 dopamine receptors) or suppressed (D_2 receptors). Natural responses to stimulation modulate discrete subpopulations of spiny neurons for normal response and behavior. Stimulants induce a sustained elevation in the extracellular dopamine and excite spiny neurons to drive aberrant behaviors.

Cocaine, amphetamines, methylphenidate, and modafinil all enhance dopamine transmission by acting on the dopamine transporters. The administration of cocaine or amphetamines increases the brain extracellular dopamine concentrations in the striatum and the nucleus accumbens. There is also an increased in the D_1 receptors in the striatum and also increased sensitivity in the nucleus accumbens. The euphoria or "high" associated with stimulants appears related to the action of the time and intensity of the stimulants in the brain with dopamine transporter occupancy and with the extracellular dopamine release in the striatum [64]. Even presentation of cues related to consumption of stimulants has been documented to enhance release of dopamine in the striatum. In vivo human studies of the brain with PET scanning show that cocaine users have decreased dopamine D_2 receptor binding in the striatum and frontal cortex while having normal levels of dopamine transporter binding [64]. Amphetamine users, in contrast, demonstrate increased D_1 receptors in the nucleus accumbens and decreased dopamine transporter density in the nucleus accumbens, striatum, and prefrontal cortex.

Cocaine, amphetamines, methylphenidate, phentermine, and ephedrine increase norepinephrine neurotransmission acting on the norepinephrine transporters. The majority of the stimulants appear to have lesser effects on the serotonin transporters with the exception of cocaine. It blocks uptake at the transporters for serotonin, dopamine, and norepinephrine at equal potency. Cocaine increases extracellular serotonin concentrations in the nucleus accumbens and VTA thereby reducing the action of the serotonin neurons in the dorsal raphe.

Endogenous opiate receptors in the brain (endorphins, enkephalins) are influenced by stimulants. Cocaine users show increased mu opiate receptor binding with PET scanning. Postmortem fatal cocaine overdoses also demonstrate kappa opiate receptor binding in the limbic area [65].

Cocaine or amphetamine both increase release of glutamate in the VTA, nucleus accumbens, dorsal striatum, ventral pallidum, septum, and cerebellum. Several of the glutamate receptors are important in the reinforcement of cocaine. Blocking NMDA in the nucleus accumbens decreases cocaine reinforcement along with reduction of mGluR5 receptor activity. Stimulation of the presynaptic mGluR2 receptors reduces cocaine reinforcement but reduction of the mGluR2 activity actually enhances reinforcement. Chronic use of cocaine may decrease nonsynaptic extracellular glutamate. Withdrawal from chronic cocaine use decreases the membrane excitability in GABA-containing spiny neurons which then induces a persistent upregulation of AMPA-glutamate receptors on the spiny neurons. This makes the spiny neurons more receptive to glutamate input from the cortex and other regions.

Cocaine and methamphetamine block neuronal nicotinic acetylcholine (Ach) receptors and cocaine also blocks the muscarinic Ach receptors in the brain and cardiac myocytes [66]. The stimulants cause Ach release in the striatum, nucleus accumbens, medial thalamus, and interpeduncular nucleus. Cocaine used chronically down-regulates the brain cholinergic systems and methamphetamine upregulates the cholinergic system.

Further research needs to be accomplished to further understand the complex and interdependent nature of the effects on receptors of addictive drugs on the brain and other organ systems.

References

1. Stepensky D. Prediction of drug disposition on the basis of its chemical structure. Clin Pharmacokinet. 2013;52:415–31.
2. Johnson F, Setnik B. Morphine sulfate and naltrexone hydrochloride extended-release capsules: naltrexone release, pharmacodynamics, and tolerability. Pain Physician. 2011;14(4):391–406.
3. Won CS, Oberlies NH, Paine MF. Mechanisms underlying food-drug interactions: inhibition of intestinal metabolism and transport. Pharmacol Ther. 2012;136:186–201.
4. Hermann R, von Richter O. Clinical evidence of herbal drugs as perpetrators of pharmacokinetic drug interactions. Planta Med. 2012;78(13):1458–77.
5. Rowland M, Tozer TN. Clinical pharmacokinetics concepts and applicants. 3rd ed. Baltimore: Lippincott Williams and Wilkins; 1995.
6. Geier EG, Schlessinger A, Fran H, et al. Structure-based ligand discovery for the Large-neutral Amino Acid Transporter 1, LAT-1. Proc Natl Acad Sci U S A. 2013;110(14):5480–5.
7. Ince I, Knibbe CA, Danhof M, et al. Development changes in the expression and function of cytochrome P450 3A isoforms: evidence from in vitro and in vivo investigations. Clin Pharmacokinet. 2013;52(5):215–33.
8. Daly AK. Genetic polymorphisms affecting drug metabolism: recent advances and clinical aspects. Adv Pharmacol. 2012;63:137–67.
9. Meyer MR, Maurer HH. Absorption, distribution, metabolism, and excretion pharmacogenomics of drugs of abuse. Pharmacogenomics. 2011;12(2):215–33.
10. Mroziewicz M, Tyndale RF. Pharmacogenetics: a tool for identifying genetic factors in drug dependence and response to treatment. Addict Sci Clin Pract. 2010;5(2):17–29.
11. Sturgess JE, George TP, Kennedy JL, et al. Pharmacogenetics of alcohol, nicotine and drug addiction treatments. Addict Biol. 2011;16(3):357–76.

12. Daly AK, Brockmoller J, Broly F, et al. Nomenclature for human CYP2D6 alleles. Pharmacogenomics. 1996;6(3):193–201.
13. Kelly LE, Madadi P. Is there a role for therapeutic drug monitoring with codeine? Ther Drug Monit. 2012;34(3):249–56.
14. Madadi P, Avard D, Koren G. Pharmacogenetics of opioids for the treatment of acute maternal pain during pregnancy and lactation. Curr Drug Metab. 2012;13(6):721–7.
15. Zhu AZX, Cox LS, Nollen N, et al. CYP2B6 and bupropion's smoking-cessation pharmacology: the role of hydroxypropion. Clin Pharmacol Ther. 2012;92(6):771–7.
16. Hung CC, Chiou MH. huang BH, et al. Impact of genetic polymorphisms in ABCB1, CYP2B6, OPRM1, ANKK1, and DRD2 genes on methadone therapy in Han Chinese patients. Pharmacogenomics. 2011;12(11):1525–33.
17. Tian JN, Ho IK, Tsou HH, et al. UGT2B7 genetic polymorphisms are associated with the withdrawal symptoms in methadone maintenance patients. Pharmacogenomics. 2012;13(8):879–88.
18. Chenowith MJ, O'Loughlin J, Sylvestre MP, et al. CYP2A6 slow nicotine metabolism is associated with increased quitting b adolescent smokers. Pharmacogenet Genomics. 2013;23(4):232–5.
19. Dutheil F, Beaune P, Loriot MA. Xenobiotic metabolizing enzymes in the central nervous system: contribution of cytochrome P450 enzymes in normal and pathological human brain. Biochimie. 2008;90(3):708–14.
20. Hedlund E, Gustafsson JA, Warner M. Cytochrome P450 in the brain: a review. Curr Drug Metab. 2001;2(3):245–63.
21. Kim JA, Bartlett S, He L, et al. Morphine induced receptor endocytosis in a novel knockin mouse reduces tolerance and dependence. Curr Biol. 2008;18(2):129–35.
22. Eiden LE, Weihe E. VMAT2: a dynamic regulator of brain monoaminergic neuronal function interacting with drugs of abuse. Ann N Y Acad Sci. 2011;1216:86–98.
23. Gilchrist A. Modulating G, protein-coupled receptors: from traditional pharmacology to allosterics. Trends Pharmacol Sci. 2007;28(8):431–7.
24. Trevor AJ, Way WL. Sedative-hypnotic drugs. In: Katzung BG, editor. Basic and clinical pharmacology. 8th ed. New York: Lange Medical Books/McGraw-Hill; 2001. p. 364–81.
25. O'Brien CP. Drug addictions and drug abuse. In: Hardman JG, Limbird LE, Gilman AG, editors. Goodman and Gilman's the pharmacologic basis of therapeutics. 10th ed. New York: McGraw-Hill; 2001. p. 621–42.

26. Garces JM, de la Torre R, Gutierrez J, et al. Clinical effectiveness of naloxone in acute ethanol intoxication. Rev Clin Esp. 1993; 193:431.
27. Vonghia L, Leggio L, Ferrulli A, et al. Acute alcohol intoxication. Eur J Intern Med. 2008;19:561.
28. Koob GF, Volkow ND. Neurocircuitry of addiction. Neuropsychopharmacology. 2009;35:217.
29. Saal D, Dong Y, Bonci A, et al. Drugs of abuse and stress trigger a common synaptic adaptation in dopamine neurons. Neuron. 2003;37:577.
30. Beckley JT, Evins CE, Fedarovich H, et al. Medical prefrontal cortex inversely regulates toluene-induced changes in markers of synaptic plasticity of mesolimbic dopamine neurons. J Neurosci. 2013;33:804.
31. Wang J, Lanfranco MF, Gibb SL, et al. Long-lasting adaptations of the NR2B-containing NMDA receptors in the dorsomedial striatum play a crucial role in alcohol consumption and relapse. J Neurosci. 2010;30:10187.
32. Sinha R, Li CS. Imaging stress-and cue-induced drug and alcohol craving; association with relapse and clinical implications. Drug Alcohol Rev. 2007;26:25.
33. Myrick H, Anton RF, Li X, et al. Differential brain activity in alcoholics and social drinkers to alcohol cues: relationship to craving. Neuropsychopharmacology. 2004;29:393.
34. Wallner M, Hancher HJ, Olsen RW. Ethanol enhances alpha 4 beta 3 delta and alpha 6 beta 3 delta gamma-aminobutyric acid type A receptors at low concentrations known to affect humans. Proc Natl Acad Sci U S A. 2003;100:15218.
35. Roberto M, Madamba SG, Moore SD, et al. Ethanol increases GABergic transmission at both pre- and postsynaptic sites in rat central amygdale neurons. Proc Natl Acad Sci U S A. 2003;100:2053.
36. Beckley JT, Joodward JJ. The abused inhalant toluene differentially modulates excitatory and inhibitory synaptic transmission in deep-layer neurons of the medial prefrontal cortex. Neuropsychopharmacology. 2011;36:1531.
37. Jin C, Smothers CT, Woodward JJ. Enhanced ethanol inhibitions of recombinant N-methyl-D-aspartate receptors by magnesium: role of NR3A subunits. Alcohol Clin Exp Res. 2008;32:1059.
38. Jin C, Woodward JJ. Effects of 8 different NR1 splice variants on the ethanol inhibition of recombinant NMDA receptors. Alcohol Clin Exp Res. 2006;30:673.

39. Tu Y, Kroener S, Abernathy K, et al. Ethanol inhibits persistent activity in prefrontal cortical neurons. J Neurosci. 2007;27:4765.
40. Dani J, Betrand D. Nicotinic acetylcholine receptors and nicotinic cholinergic mechanisms of the central nervous system. Annu Rev Pharmacol Toxicol. 2007;4:699.
41. Khakh BS, North RA. Neuromodulation by extracellular ATP and P2X receptors in the CNS. Neuron. 2012;76:51.
42. Brodie MS, Pesold C, Appel SB. Ethanol directly excites dopaminergic ventral tegmental area reward neurons. Alcohol Clin Exp Res. 1999;23:1848.
43. Oswald LM, Wand GS. Opioids and alcoholism. Physiol Behav. 2004;81:339.
44. Pava MJ, Woodward JJ. A review of the interactions between alcohol and the endocannabinoid system: implications for alcohol dependence and future directions for research. Alcohol. 2012;46:185.
45. Drover DR. Comparative pharmacokinetics and pharmacodynamics of short-acting hyposedatives: zaleplon, zolpidem, and zopiclone. Clin Pharmacokinet. 2004;43(4):227–38.
46. Fleck MW. Molecular actions of (S)-desmethylzopiclone (SEP-174559), an anxiolytic metabolite of zopiclone. J Pharmacol Exp Ther. 2002;302(2):612–8.
47. Sanna E, Busonero F, Talani G, et al. Comparison of the effects of zaleplon, zolpidem, and triazolam at various GABA(A) receptor subtypes. Eur J Pharmacol. 2002;451(2):103–10.
48. Mandrioli R, Mercolini L, Raggi MA. Metabolism of benzodiazepine and non-benzodiazepine anxiolytic-hypnotic drugs: an analytical point of view. Curr Drug Metab. 2010;11(9):815–29.
49. Beanarroch EE. GABAA receptor heterogeneity, function, and implications for epilepsy. Neurology. 2007;68(8):612–4.
50. Lingford-Hughes A, Hume SP, Feeney A, et al. Imaging the GABA-benzodiazepine receptor subtype containing the alpha5-subunit in vivo with [11C]Ro154513 positron emission tomography. J Cereb Blood Flow Metab. 2002;22(7):878–89.
51. McKernan RM, Rosaahl TW, Reynolds DS, et al. Sedative but not anxiolytic properties of benzodiazepines are mediated by the GABA(A) receptor alpha 1 subtype. Nat Neurol. 2000;3(6):587–92.
52. Dias R, Shepard WF, Fradley RL, et al. Evidence for a significant role of alpha 3-containing GABA-A receptors in mediating the anxiolytic effects of benzodiazepines. J Neurosci. 2005;25(46):10682–8.

53. Gutstein H, Akil H. Opioid analgesics. In: Brunton L, Lazo L, Parker K, editors. Goodman and Gillman's the pharmacological basis of therapeutics. 11th ed. New York: McGraw-Hill; 2005. p. 547–90.
54. Raynor K, Kong H, Mestek A, et al. Characterization of the cloned human mu opioid receptor. J Pharmacol Exp Ther. 1995;272:423–8.
55. Inturrisi CE. Clinical pharmacology of opioids for pain. Clin J Pain. 2002;18:S1–13.
56. Ferrari A, Coccia CP, Bertolini A, et al. Methadone-metabolism, pharmacokinetics and interactions. Pharmacol Res. 2004;50: 551–9.
57. Kobayashi K, Yamamoteo T, Chiba K, et al. Human buprenorphine N-dealkylation is catalyzed by cytochrome P450 3a4. Drug Metab Dispos. 1998;26:818–21.
58. Fleckenstein AE, Gibb JW, Hanson GR. Differential effects of stimulants on monoaminergic transporters: pharmacological consequences and implications for neurotoxicity. Eur J Pharmacol. 2000;406:1–13.
59. Telang FW, Volkow ND, Levy A, et al. Distribution of tracer levels of cocaine in the human brain as assessed with averaged [11C] cocaine images. Synapse. 1993;31:290–6.
60. Cone EJ. Pharmacokinetics and pharmacodynamics of cocaine. J Anal Toxicol. 1995;19:459–78.
61. Warner A, Norman AB. Mechanisms of cocaine hydrolysis and metabolism in vitro and in vivo: a clarification. Ther Drug Monit. 2000;22:266–70.
62. Maurer HH, Sauer C, Theobald DS. Toxicokinetics of drugs of abuse: current knowledge of the isozymes involved in the human metabolism of tetrahydrocannabinol, cocaine, heroin, morphine, and codeine. Ther Drug Monit. 2006;28:447–53.
63. Feltenstein MW. The neurocircuitry of addiction: an overview. Br J Pharmacol. 2008;154:261–74.
64. Volkow ND, Fowler JS, Wang GJ, et al. Imaging dopamine's role in drug abuse and addiction. Neuropharmacology. 2009;56 Suppl 1:3–8.
65. Staley JK, Rothman RB, Rice KC, et al. K_2 opioid receptors in limbic area of the human brain are upregulated by cocaine in fatal overdose victims. J Neurosci. 1997;17:8225–33.
66. Williams MJ, Adinoff B. The role of acetylcholine in cocaine addiction. Neuropsychopharmacology. 2008;33:1779–97.

Chapter 4
Women's Specific Issues in Addiction

Denise Burgess

A myth exists in the world of women's fashions called "one size fits all." Every woman alive knows there is no article of clothing that will truly fit all sizes. Sadly, the approach to the treatment of addictions has historically been a "one size fits all" approach. The opportunity exists to recognize the unique circumstances of women dealing with addiction issues and the treatment modalities that will most effectively treat their disease. The motivation needed to move women towards recovery as well as the approach to treatment differs from that of men [1]. Recognizing these differences and directing care appropriately is a competency to be embraced by all providers.

Despite progress of the Women's movement a gender bias persists in Western culture. The role of nurturer continues to be perceived primarily as that of the female's responsibility. This bias transfers to the stigma women with addiction issues experience. The mantra is that because a female has potential to procreate, the capacity to nurture should/could protect women from engaging in behaviors that are counterintuitive to nurturing. Traditional households where the women

D. Burgess, RN, BSN, MA, LPC, NBCC (✉)
Charleston Area Medical Center, Charleston, WV, USA
e-mail: denise.burgess@camc.org

© Springer International Publishing Switzerland 2016
B.C. Calhoun, T. Lewis (eds.), *Tobacco Cessation and Substance Abuse Treatment in Women's Healthcare*,
DOI 10.1007/978-3-319-26710-4_4

continue to be the primary caretakers of children will perpetuate these stereotypes [2]. As much as the glass ceiling has been pushed and the percentage of "June Cleaver's" home vacuuming in her pearls has been replaced with significant numbers of professional women, the stereotype persists that the female is responsible for familial unity and sustainment of all things protective.

The state of Tennessee's legislation in 2013 making it possible for a woman to be charged with aggravated assault if she tests positive for drugs during her pregnancy is being debated heavily in the literature as discriminatory and showing little insight into the complexity of substance abuse [3].

These beliefs perpetuate the shame that women feel and exacerbates the secrecy and hesitancy to seek treatment thus resulting in lower numbers of women engaged in recovery [4]. The result is that women find creative ways to hide their substance use and when at long last they are confronted, they often fail to disclose. Women too can discriminate against other women in this same manner. Pregnant women attending AA or NA meetings have found themselves shunned. Belittling comments even amongst the recovery community have differentiated the recovering addict from the "bottom feeding" addict who will use even though she's pregnant [5].

A woman willing to engage in treatment often is met with substantial barriers that may tax her already poor distress tolerance skills and reinforce her perception of failure. Historically, the large percentage of women working in service line business and industry have been employed by companies that offer minimal to no benefits. Even with the passing of the mental health parity law in 2008 discrimination against mental health and substance abuse issues has persisted.

The scheduled times of 12-step meetings, lack of child care at meetings or for appointments with mental health and substance abuse professionals and geographic constraints, and transportation issues are all potential barriers for women receiving treatment. A lack of public service information regarding the resources for treatment, coupled with the shame and stigma described previously, compile the roadblocks for women desiring help [6].

The distinct correlation between women suffering from addiction issues and those living as victims of intimate partner violence is well documented. Controlling partners and partners who have substance abuse issues themselves can prevent women from seeking treatment. The absence of intimate partners, the partner's level of drug or alcohol use, and the heightened anxiety experienced in the family system in the absence of the female who is participating in treatment are found to be influential in the decision to seek help by the woman with substance abuse issues [4].

Chapter 4

An ongoing debate exists amongst providers regarding the most effective treatment approaches for clients dealing with addiction issues. Time demands, philosophical approaches, organizational hierarchies, and provider bias all have the potential to impact the method of treatment that will be applied. When self-disclosure and screening questionnaires are stand-alone tools for diagnosing substance abuse issues, a high percentage of at risk patients will be missed [1]. Recognizing cues, discrepancies, and early warning signs of substance abuse has become a crucial skill of the effective, thorough diagnostician.

The clinician, who desires to be thorough in identifying and treating the female patient effectively, must be aware of their own biases and preconceived notions. A patient seeking treatment that appears affluent or well educated is less likely to be considered as someone with a potential addiction issue [2]. Use of universal drug and alcohol screening in private practice is much less prevalent than that in clinic-based practices. In part this has contributed to the false assumption that the more influential, financially stable, or well educated a patient is, the more unlikely it is that she will be engaged in illicit activities.

The use of validating messages can be a first step towards building a therapeutic relationship with the female client struggling with substance issues. If the school of thought that the substance abuse is symptomatic of larger issues is correct, identifying and treating those issues, most notably, a history of trauma is imperative if intervention is going to be effective [3]. The female client who has never developed a sense of self, or who has surrendered that sense of self due to abuse or neglect; who has little to no concept of belonging and who has had few opportunities for success, are going to find treatment interventions overwhelming. Something as simple as referring to a "class" they need to attend may conjure up images of school failure that the client has experienced and thus sabotage treatment before it's begun.

Considering the individual needs of the client and designing intervention accordingly will promote the greatest opportunity for success. Assessing the educational level of the patient, her distress tolerance and coping skills, social situation, economic factors, and support systems should be considered when creating a treatment plan for women with substance abuse issues.

The utilization of Motivational Interviewing has increased significantly in the area of substance abuse treatment over the past decade. The premise of MI is that by appealing to the client's intrinsic motivation the clinician will guide the client to the desired change. Reflective listening, the use of affirmations and eliciting from the client, and goals that she would wish to accomplish are tools of MI that are believed to help accomplish sobriety [4].

Traditional 12-step programs such as Alcoholics Anonymous and Narcotics Anonymous have been recommended in the addictions world for years. The philosophy of the 12-step programs is that by utilizing support groups, adopting and "working" the various steps of the program and abstaining from all use of alcohol or drugs the participant will be "in recovery." The belief is that one is never "recovered" from the addiction, but rather must persist in these behavioral changes to continue to "recover" [5].

Cognitive Behavioral Therapy, a model of therapy that examines the relationship between the client's thoughts, feelings, and behaviors is also the foundation of numerous treatment programs for substance abuse issues. By changing her thought from, "I am a victim to my disease of drug abuse," to "I can choose to overcome my drug abuse," the client can change her feelings from that of victim to that of someone who is empowered and thus change behavior and become clean or sober. Opponents of these concepts will argue that disbelief in free-will disrupts the CBT potential and addicts will use this as a scapegoat for needing to control their own destiny [6].

An emerging thought in the treatment of addictions is to neither dismiss the disease model vs. free will debate but to recognize that there exists a shared governance. Rather than viewing addiction as a disease where a patient's predisposition or chemical makeup dooms them to a world of abusing drugs and alcohol, that addiction is viewed similarly to Type II Diabetes. A client's choices may still influence whether they develop an addiction by the behavior in which they choose to engage [7].

Dialectical Behavior Therapy, a form of Cognitive Behavioral Therapy was introduced in the late 1980s as a treatment for clients with Axis II Diagnoses, primarily Borderline Personality Disorder. As the psychotherapy began displaying positive results in this patient population, transference of the concepts to other psychiatric illnesses, including addiction, was implemented. Consistent success has been demonstrated using DBT for the treatment of women with drug dependence [8]. The structure and reinforcement of the DBT model provides a community to the recovering woman that models healthy communication and social dynamics that may be unknown to them outside the treatment arena.

Contingency management or incentive programs have been supported in emerging evidence as an effective approach to the treatment of women suffering from addiction. This approach is seen as a way to facilitate recovery and provide a positive experience for the patient [9]. Clients participating in such programs articulate positive responses when interviewed regarding their perceptions of the incentive program. Likewise, acceptance by the provider of the concept of contingency management appears to have an impact on the outcome [10].

A relatively new approach to treatment is that of incorporating a realization of one's health—an intrinsic connection to health and wellness—into the treatment model. Coined Health Realization the goal is to teach the client a set of principles that focuses on the understanding of the principles of Consciousness, Thought, and Mind from a model developed by Mills and Pransky. Rather than focusing on disorders or disease models, Health Realization which has been used in other arenas for over 30 years, has been incorporated into substance abuse programs to reduce depression and anxiety and improve personal relationships and improved self-esteem [11]. This model has been used primarily in inpatient treatment models and thus consideration for a client needing an outpatient modality of treatment should be directed to a therapist or mental health professional who has specific credentials in this treatment methodology.

Regardless of the treatment model selected for female clients, the literature repeatedly supports that the interventions that approach the patient's treatment from a systemic model are the most effective. Involving the client's family, community, or identified source of support in treatment provides the link and validation that are significant to female clients [12]. Furthermore, the interaction with other women facing the same crisis is also believed to be a guiding principle in successful treatment [13].

There is no "one size fits all" and the clinician must invest time to connect with the client to determine a modality that is most suited for that client. Utilizing multidisciplinary team approaches to the client's treatment provides the clinician with a multitude of resources to hopefully treat the client holistically. It cannot be emphasized enough that diagnosing and providing treatment for client's with a history of trauma is crucial to positive outcomes. Otherwise, only the symptoms are being addressed and we have failed to reach the core of the patient's need.

Lastly, awareness of one's own biases in the treatment of the female patient suffering from addiction or substance abuse issues is warranted. Because addictions affect such a significant percentage of people, it is likely that the provider has personal experience either directly or indirectly with someone suffering from a dependency or addictive disorder. Differentiating personal feelings from professional judgment can become difficult if the provider has not processed through their own issues with addiction. This becomes compounded further when the addict is a woman because it again is in conflict with our stereotype of females as the nurturers of our society. This bias does not bypass female providers. Counterproductive attitudes of female providers have been documented to impede effective treatment of the client [1].

The National Institutes of Health estimated in the beginning of the new millennium that of the 294 billion estimated cost of substance abuse, 12 billion dollars a year is spent on the treatment of addictions [14]. Though that amount is a statistically small percentage of the estimated cost given the high incidence of recidivism, the question exists of how effective is our approach. While this debate is likely to go on for decades, one statistic is irrefutable; not providing any treatment or intervention will lead to even greater health care issues and a continued threat to our public health. We have a unique opportunity in treating women to attempt to steer them towards a model of health and wellness that will ultimately impact their family and community. Providers can no longer ignore the issue of substance abuse and addiction amongst their patients. They have a duty and obligation to educate themselves about effective treatment options and in a nonjudgmental, compassionate manner work with their patients to create an effective treatment plan.

References Chapter 4

1. Williams K. Attitudes of mental health professionals to co-morbidity between mental health problems and substance misuse. J Ment Health. 1999;8(6):605–13.
2. Lewandowski C, Hill T. The impact of emotional and material social support on women's drug treatment completion. Health Soc Work. 2009;34(3):213–21.

3. Anderson S. A critical analysis of the concept of codependency. Soc Work. 1994;39(6):677–84.

4. http://sbirt.samhsa.gov.

5. Bry B. Preventing substance abuse by supporting families' efforts with community resources. Child Family Behav Ther. 1994;16:21–6.

6. Vohs KD, Schooler JW. The value of believing in free will: encouraging a belief in determinism increases cheating. Psychol Sci. 2008;19:49–54.

7. Kathleen Vohs & Roby Baumeister Addiction Research & Theory, June 2009;17(3):231–5.

8. Linehan M, Schmidt H, Dimeff L, et al. Dialectical behavior therapy for patients with borderline personality disorder and drug-dependence. Am J Addict. 1999;8:279–92.

9. Weinstock J, Alessi SM, Petry NM. Regardless of psychiatric severity the addition of contingency management to standard treatment improves retention and drug use outcomes. Drug Alcohol Depend. 2007;87:288–96.

10. Srebnik D, Sugar A, Coblentz P, et al. Acceptability of contingency management among clinicians and clients within a co-occurring mental health and substance use treatment program. Am J Addict. 2013;22:432–6.

11. Pransky G, Mills R, Sedgeman J, et al. An emerging paradigm for brief treatment and prevention. In: Vandercreek L, Knapp S, Jackson T, editors. Innovations in clinical practice: a source book, vol. 15. Sarasota: Professional Resource Press; 1997. p. 76–98.

12. Wasserman DA, Stewart AL, Delucchi KL. Social support and abstinence from opiates and cocaine during opioid maintenance treatment. Drug Alcohol Depend. 2001;66:65–75.

13. Stanton D, Todd T, & Associates. The family therapy of drug abuse and addiction. New York: Guilford; 1982.

14. http://www.ncbi.nlm.nih.gov/pmc/articles/PMC1402649/.

Chapter 5
Health Effects

Byron C. Calhoun

Tobacco

Tobacco abuse is the leading cause of death in the United States [1–3]. It is linked to some 440,000 deaths a year with some $100 billion in direct medical costs and nearly $100 billion in lost productivity annually [4]. There have been estimates made that each pack of cigarettes costs an estimated $7.18 in medical care and lost work [5]. Cigarettes increase the risk of developing and amplify respiratory tract infections, influenza, pneumococcal pneumonia, and TB. It has been estimated that adult men lose 13.2 years of life and adult women 14.5 years of life as a result of tobacco abuse. There have also been estimates of passive smoking attributable to some 40,000 deaths, with 35,000 due to cardiovascular disease, 3000 from lung cancer, and some 1000 from perinatal issues [5].

Tobacco consists of volatile and particulate states that contain multiple substances other than nicotine that are responsible for morbidity and mortality. The volatile state

B.C. Calhoun, MD, FACOG, FACS, FASAM, MBA (✉)
Department of Obstetrics and Gynecology, West Virginia
University-Charleston, Charleston, WV, USA
e-mail: Byron.calhoun@camc.org

© Springer International Publishing Switzerland 2016   83
B.C. Calhoun, T. Lewis (eds.), *Tobacco Cessation and
Substance Abuse Treatment in Women's Healthcare*,
DOI 10.1007/978-3-319-26710-4_5

contains over 500 gaseous compounds that include: nitrogen, CO, carbon dioxide, ammonia, hydrogen cyanide, and benzene. There are also more than 3500 different compounds in the particulate state consisting of active alkaloids nornicotine, anabasine, anatabine, myosmine, nicotyrine, and nicotine. The tar of the cigarette is the particulate matter minus the alkaloid and water portion. The tar of the cigarette contains the carcinogens of aromatic hydrocarbons, N-nitrosamines, and aromatic amines.

With smoking there over 4000 different chemicals released including some 50 known carcinogens. The increased risk of cardiovascular disease is related to the oxidant chemical exposure and CO along with hydrogen cyanide, carbon disulfide, cadmium, and zinc [6]. Chronic obstructive lung disease appears related to exposure to tar, nitrogen oxide, hydrogen cyanide, and volatile aldehydes. This oxidative stress causes the generation of superoxide radicals and hydrogen peroxide with lung damage. The most significant contribution to lung cancers appears to be the polynuclear aromatic hydrocarbons and tobacco N-nitrosamines with polonium-210 and the volatile aldehydes. Catechol, volatile aldehydes, and nitrogen oxide all increase the formation of N-nitrosamines which are linked to tumorigenesis. The risk of oral, larynx, esophagus, lung, stomach, pancreas, kidney, urinary bladder, uterine cervix, and leukemia are related to the intensity and duration of cigarette smoking. Cigarette smoking also causes skin changes with increased risk of skin cancers, wrinkling, and premature aging of the skin. There have also been links to cataracts and possibly macular degeneration as well. Women who smoke also demonstrate lower estrogen levels with earlier menopause and osteoporosis. In males, smoking may impair penile erection and doubles the likelihood of erectile dysfunction.

Nicotine suppresses appetite and smokers weigh 2.7–4.5 kg less than non-smokers. Nicotine also increases lipolysis and the release of free fatty acids in liver. This may contribute to the decrease in high-density lipoproteins seen in smokers. Smoking is also linked to delayed healing of peptic ulcers with decreased production of endogenous prostaglandins and decrease in the mucous bicarbonate barrier in the stomach.

In summary, tobacco has been linked to the following cardiovascular effects: atherosclerosis, stroke, myocardial infarction, peripheral vascular disease, corpulmonale, erectile dysfunction, hypertension control issues, angina, and dysrhythmias; renal effects: renal failure and hypertension; gastrointestinal effects: peptic ulcers, gastroesophageal reflux, malignancy of stomach and pancreas; pulmonary effects: lung cancer, chronic obstructive lung disease, reactive airway, pneumonia, bronchitis, pulmonary hypertension, interstitial lung disease, and pneumothorax; neurologic effects: stroke, small-vessel ischemia, and cognitive deficits; infectious disease: bronchitis, pneumonia, upper respiratory tract infection; sleep effects: insomnia and increased sleep latency; trauma effects; burns and smoke inhalation; perioperative effects: pulmonary infection, difficulty weaning off ventilators/oxygen, respiratory failure, and reactive airway exacerbations; hematologic effects: hypercoagulability; musculoskeletal: compartment syndromes and fractures; and nutritional lacks.

Marijuana

Marijuana affects several psychomotor functions in a dose-dependent manner including object distance, shape discrimination, reaction time, information processing, perceptual motor coordination, motor performance, signal detection, tracking behaviors, and slowed time perception [7]. Marijuana particularly affects to a greater extent those tasks that are more complex requiring sustained concentration. There is an additive effect to cannabis with alcohol especially with driving.

Cannabis usage has been linked to "amotivational syndrome" with lack of initiative and decreased executive function. Some authors point to possible confounders with alcohol use, other substances, and social surroundings. It is clear from the scientific literature that adolescent substance abusers suffer from attention, memory, and executive function deficits [8]. Baa and Tapert, 2010 note in their review of the substance body of literature noting alterations in the prefrontal, hippocampal, cerebellar structure and function as well as white matter structural integrity [8]. In line with this there are the subtle decreases in intellectual function and memory, attention, and integration of complicated information. Complex reaction times, perception, reading, arithmetic performance, recall, and memory appear affected as well. One 20-year prospective study found that heavy users lost IQ points (average 6) while nonusers gained (average 1 point) [9]. Further, the persistent users had significant loss in learning, memory, and executive decision making [9].

Effects on major organ systems are also found. The major health effect appears to be the damage to the respiratory system since many of the same carcinogens found in tobacco are also found in marijuana smoke. Marijuana smoking increases airway resistance, decreases pulmonary function, produces chronic cough, airway inflammation, and atypical cell growth. There has not been enough data available at this time to link marijuana to lung cancer. Marijuana appears to suppress macrophage function and natural killer cell activity thus impairing host resistance to infections. Marijuana increases heart rate and produces orthostatic hypotension which are of little effects in healthy young adults but may be significant in older users.

Cannabinoid receptors are significant actors in the development of a variety of liver pathology. The chronic use of THC appears to increase steatosis with increased live fibrosis. There is also inhibition of liver microsomes with prolongation of certain medications (i.e., barbiturates). Renal complications appear only rarely. The effects on the endocrine are significant that virtually every system is affected in some way. THC effects include: inhibition of pituitary luteinizing hormone, prolactin, and growth hormone. The effects on the human thyroid are not well documented. THC use may affect female reproduction including production of galactorrhea.

Marijuana may produce euphoria, hunger, and possible relaxation. There have also been reports of panic, anxiety, nausea, and dizziness. These effects are more likely with oral doses of 20 mg or more in a naïve user.

Hallucinogens

This includes the chemical substances that alter cognitive, perceptual, and emotional understanding of reality and self. These include classical hallucinogens (mescaline, psilocybin, LSD, dimethyltryptamine); the entactogenic phenylalkylamines (methylenedioxyamphetamine, MDMA, MDE); anticholinergic dissociatives (atropine, hyoscyamine, scopolamine); and dissociative anesthetics (phencyclidine [PCP], ketamine, salvinorin A). Physical effects include mild effects: tachycardia, palpitations, slight hypo or hypertension, diaphoresis, slight hyperthermia, motor incoordination, tremor, hyperreflexia, and altered neuroendocrine functioning; mild to strong physical effects: mydriasis, arousal, and insomnia; and rare physical effects: nausea, vomiting, diarrhea, blurred vision, nystagmus, piloerection, and salivation. Psychological effects include typical effects: intensification and lability of affect with euphoria, anxiety, depression, and/or cathartic expressions, dream state, sensory activation with illusion, pseudohallucinations, hallucinations, and/or synesthesia, altered experience of time and space, altered body image, increased suggestibility, lassitude/indifference/detachment, acute cognitive alterations with loosening of association, inability for goal-directed thinking, and memory disturbance; "positive" psychological effects include: sense of perceiving deeper layers of the world, oneself, and others, mystical experience, and sense of profound discovery/healing; and "negative" psychological effects include: psychosomatic complaints, impaired judgement, derealization, depersonalization, megalomania, impulsivity, odd behaviors, paranoid delusions, and suicidal ideation. The national survey by the National Survey on Drug Use and Health (NSDUH) in 2010 estimated that about 37.5 million (14.8 %) Americans over age 12 years used a hallucinogen at least once in their lifetime [10]. In conclusion, hallucinogens are a heterogeneous class of drugs with diverse effects and mechanisms of action. They are physiologically non-toxic in medium doses with main complications resulting from unsupervised use.

Disassociatives

Drugs act as antagonists of the N-methyl-D-aspartate (NMDA) receptor subtypes of the major excitatory neurotransmitter, glutamic acid, of the brain. This includes phencyclidine (PCP), ketamine dizocilpine, dextromethorphan (DXM), and nitrous oxide. The clinical effects are the dissociative state of intoxication. The major effects are impairments in working and episodic memory along with cognitive task problems. PCP may cause an acute reaction similar to catatonic schizophrenia. PCP may also induce an organic brain syndrome along with cardiovascular and renal toxicity. DXM abuse may cause brain damage, seizures, loss of consciousness, irregular heart rate, and even death. It may even cause respiratory depression.

Alcohol

Alcohol affects all tissue and organ systems and in heavy drinkers there is skeletal fragility, brain/liver/heart damage and susceptibility to cancers. Moderate alcohol use (<2 drinks per day) have been associated with some benefits, including decreased risk of coronary artery disease.

In summary, alcohol has been linked to the following cardiovascular effects: cardiomyopathy, atrial fibrillation (holiday heart), hypertension, dysrhythmia, masking angina symptoms, coronary artery spasm, myocardial ischemia, high-output states, coronary artery disease, and sudden death; liver effects: steatosis (fatty liver), acute and chronic hepatitis infection [B or C] or toxic [acetaminophen], alcoholic hepatitis, cirrhosis, portal hypertension and varices, spontaneous bacterial peritonitis; renal effects: hepatorenal syndrome, rhabdomyolysis and acute renal failure, volume depletion and prerenal failure, acidosis, hypokalemia, hypophosphatemia; gastrointestinal effects: gastritis, pancreatitis, diarrhea, malabsorption (pancreatic insufficiency or folate/lactase deficiency, parotid enlargement, malignancy, colitis, Barrett's esophagus, gastroesophageal reflux, Mallory-Weiss syndrome, and GI bleeding; pulmonary: aspiration, sleep apnea, respiratory depression, apnea, chemical or infectious pneumonitis; neurologic effects: peripheral and autonomic neuropathy, seizure, hepatic encephalopathy, Korsakoff dementia, Wernicke syndrome, cerebellar dysfunction, Marchiafava–Bignami syndrome, central pontine myelinolysis, myopathy, amblyopia, stroke, withdrawal delirium, hallucinations, toxic leukoencephalopathy, subdural hematoma, intracranial hemorrhage; infectious problems: Hepatitis C, pneumonia, TB, HIV, sexually transmitted diseases, spontaneous bacterial peritonitis, brain abscess, and meningitis; sleep effects: apnea, periodic limb movements of sleep, insomnia, disrupted sleep, daytime fatigue; trauma: MVA's fatal and nonfatal injuries, physical and sexual abuse; perioperative issues: withdrawal, perioperative complications (delirium, infection, bleeding, pneumonia, delayed wound healing, dysrhythmia), hepatic decompensation, hepatorenal syndrome, and death; hematologic effects include: macrocytic anemia, pancytopenia due to marrow toxicity and or splenic sequestration, leucopenia, thrombocytopenia, coagulopathy because of liver disease, iron deficiency anemia, folate deficiency, spur cell anemia, and burr cell anemia; musculoskeletal effects include: rhabdomyolysis, compartment syndromes, gout, saturnine gout, fracture, osteopenia, osteonecrosis; and nutritional effects including vitamin and mineral deficiencies (B vitamins, riboflavin, niacin, vitamin D, magnesium, calcium, folate, phosphate, and zinc).

Nonalcohol Sedative Hypnotics

These drugs include the benzodiazepines, nonbenzodiazepine hypnotics, barbiturates, and related compounds. These compounds produce effects from sedation to frank obtundation. The barbiturates are the most risk for respiratory depression. Benzodiazepine toxicity usually includes an impaired gag reflex and ataxia. Benzodiazepines withdrawal varies based upon length of administration. Short periods of use will have mild anxiety, headache, insomnia, dysphoria, tremor, and muscle twitching. Chronic long-term use may lead to autonomic dysfunction, nausea, vomiting, depersonalization, derealization, delirium, hallucinations, illusions, agitation, and grand mal seizures. Barbiturate withdrawal with acute discontinuation may lead to apprehension, uneasiness, muscular weakness, coarse tremors, postural hypotension, anorexia, vomiting, and myoclonic jerks that may last for up to 2 weeks. Grand mal seizures may occur within 2–3 days of stopping barbiturates and last for up to 8 days and delirium develops 3–8 days and may last up to 2 weeks.

Opioids

Medical complications of opioids include central nervous system, pulmonary, cardiovascular, gastrointestinal, renal, musculoskeletal, and infectious diseases. The central effects of the opioids are well-known with the overdosing of the medications varying from mild sedation to coma. Along with this effect is the suppression of the gag reflex with subsequent aspiration of stomach contents with the centrally mediated nausea and vomiting. Overdosing of opioids results in the central depression of respiration but also may lead to non-cardiogenic pulmonary edema (NCPE) with bronchospasm. NCPE presents with frothy, pick bronchial secretions, cyanosis, and rales. It is most commonly associated with intravenous or inhalational use of heroin. Cardiovascular effects usually result from the hypoxia due to respiratory depression. Opioids are thought to cause a release of histamine with vasodilation with subsequent orthostatic hypotension. Propoxyphene may cause direct myocardial toxicity. Further, high doses of methadone (>300 mg/day) have been linked to prolongation of the QT interval with torsades de pointes [11]. Gastrointestinal effects include nausea and vomiting, slowing of GI motility with constipation and possible fecal impaction. Morphine may also cause spasm of sphincter of Oddi and should not be used in biliary colic. Renal effects include rare cases of rhabdomyolysis with heroin, illicit methadone, and propoxyphene. Heroin, morphine, and pentazocine have been liked to nephropathy when used intravenously with subsequent glomerulonephritis. High doses of opioids may induce centrally mediated muscle rigidity of the chest and abdominal wall. Intravenous use may also lead to osteomyelitis, septic arthritis, polymyositis, and fibrous myopathy. Well-known infectious complications from intravenous abuse with needle sharing include HIV, hepatitis B, hepatitis C, and bacterial infections.

In summary, opioids have been linked to the following liver effects: granulomatosis; kidney effects: rhabdomyolysis, acute renal failure, and factitious hematuria; gastrointestinal effects: constipation, ileus, and intestinal pseudoobstruction; pulmonary complications: respiratory depression/failure, emphysema, bronchospasm, exacerbation of sleep apnea, and pulmonary edema; neurologic effects: seizure (overdose) and compression neuropathy; infectious complications: aspiration pneumonia; sleep problems: insomnia; trauma: MVAs and other accidental death; perioperative complications: withdrawal and problems with pain control; and musculoskeletal which includes osteopenia.

Cocaine, Amphetamines, and Other Stimulants

These compounds include the naturally occurring plant alkaloids including cocaine, ephedra, khat, and synthetic compounds such as amphetamines and methylphenidate. Virtually, all systems of the body are affected by stimulants.

Adverse neurologic effects consist of dysphoric effects like anxiety, irritability, panic attacks, interpersonal sensitivity, hypervigilance, suspiciousness, paranoia, grandiosity, impaired judgment, and psychotic symptoms like delusions and hallucinations. The stimulant psychosis may resemble acute schizophrenia. Hallucinations may be auditory, visual, somatosensory (tactile sensation of "skin crawling"). Physiologic effects may include tachycardia, dilated pupils, diaphoresis, and nausea. Chronic cocaine use may result in cognitive impairment that persists for several months after last use. Amphetamine abuse may lead to persistent paranoia and hallucinations that may last for several years. There have been psychotic flash-backs seen in methamphetamine abusers up to 2 years after last use. Cocaine and amphetamine abuse have been linked to cerebral vasoconstriction, cerebrovascular atherosclerosis, cerebrovascular disease, and strokes [12]. There are also a number of movement disorders found with stimulant abuse. These include: repetitive stereotyped behaviors (such as repeated dismantling of objects, cleaning, doodling, and searching for imaginary objects), acute dystonic reactions, choreoathetosis, and akathisa ("crack dancers"), buccolingual dyskinesias ("twisted mouth"), exacerbation of Tourette syndrome, and tardive dyskinesia.

Stimulants have direct and central nervous system effects. The direct effects include increasing adrenergic activity at sympathetic nerve terminals and in the CNS increasing heart rate, blood pressure, and systemic vascular resistance. Cocaine-induced tachycardia results in an increased oxygen demand with decreased blood flow may cause acute myocardial infarction even in a young person even without atherosclerosis. Cocaine also increases activated platelets, platelet aggregation, and thromboxane synthesis. Cocaine use has been attributed to about 25 % of nonfatal heart attacks in patients younger than 45 years of age [13]. Frequent cocaine users are up to seven times more likely to have a nonfatal heart attack than nonusers [13]. Cocaine is also associated with cardiac arrhythmias including ventricular tachycardia or ventricular fibrillation as well as sudden death. Chronic cocaine or amphetamine use is further associated with cardiomyopathy and myocarditis [14]. Cocaine-associated cases of dilated cardiomyopathy and myocardial fibrosis may be due to direct toxic effects of high concentrations of circulating norepinephrine. Cocaine-associated myocarditis may be a direct toxic effect of cocaine or hypersensitivity effect.

The effects of smoked cocaine cause both acute and chronic pulmonary toxicity [15]. Acute respiratory symptoms may develop in up to half of users within minutes to several hours after smoking. Symptoms include productive cough, shortness of breath, wheezing, chest pain, hemoptysis, and exacerbation of asthma. Severe effects include pulmonary edema, pulmonary hemorrhage, pneumothorax, pneumomediastinum, and thermal airway injury. Pulmonary edema has been reported after intravenous cocaine use. Chronic use may lead to interstitial pneumonitis and bronchiolitis obliterans.

Stimulants have no direct toxic effects on the kidneys. Acute renal failure may occur from renal ischemia or infarction, malignant hypertension, or rhabdomyolysis. Intrarenal artery constriction may cause medullary ischemia and renal tubular damage.

Cocaine reduces gastric motility and delays gastric emptying with effects on the medullary centers controlling these functions. The most serious effects of cocaine use are due to vasoconstriction and ischemia: gastroduodenal ulceration and perforation, intestinal infarction, and perforation, and ischemic colitis. Ulceration is found in the greater curvature and prepyloric region of the stomach, pyloric canal, and first portion of the duodenum. Cocaine is hepatotoxic due to the oxidative metabolism to norcocaine by the cytochrome P450 microsomal enzyme system in the liver with further changes in the hepatotoxic compound of N-hyroxynorcocaine.

Cocaine use activates the hypothalamic–pituitary–adrenal (HPA) center, stimulating the secretion of epinephrine, adrenocorticotropin releasing hormone, adrenocorticotrophic hormone (ACTH), and cortisol. Prolactin is decreased in acute cocaine use as well. Chronic cocaine has normal, increased, or decreased prolactin levels. Acute cocaine also increases plasma luteinizing hormone. Chronic cocaine users have normal testosterone, cortisol, luteinizing hormone, and thyroid hormones.

Stimulants may cause rhabdomyolysis by several mechanisms: a direct toxic effect causing myofibrillar degeneration, indirectly by vasoconstriction of intramuscular arteries resulting in ischemia, and secondary to stimulant-induced hyperthermia or seizures. Some one-third of patients with rhabdomyolysis will develop acute renal failure with occasional DIC and liver damage.

Head and neck problems with cocaine use are dependent on the route of administration. Intranasal cocaine is associated with chronic rhinitis, perforated nasal septum and nasal collapse, oropharyngeal ulcers, and osteolytic sinusitis due to vasoconstriction and necrosis. Oral cocaine is associated with gingival ulceration and erosion of dental enamel. Both cocaine and methamphetamine reduce salivary secretions and causes bruxism. Chronic use causes caries, cracking of enamel, and loss of teeth.

Cocaine has been linked with several vasculitic syndromes usually affecting skin and muscle. They may mimic Henoch–Schönlein purpura, Stevens–Johnson syndrome, or Raynaud phenomenon. Cocaine impairs the response of monocytes to bacterial infection (lipopolysaccharides).

Cocaine with chronic use reduces libido and impairs sexual function. Men may experience erectile dysfunction or delayed or inhibited ejaculation. Cocaine has been applied to the penis or clitoris as a local anesthetic effect to delay orgasm.

In summary, cocaine has been linked to the following cardiovascular effects: hypertension, myocardial infarction, angina, chest pain, supraventricular tachycardia, ventricular dysrhythmias, cardiomyopathy, myocarditis, sudden death, and aortic dissection; liver effects include ischemic necrosis and hepatitis; kidney issues include: rhabdomyolysis, acute renal failure, vasculitis, necrotizing angiitis, accelerated hypertension, nephrosclerosis, and ischemia; gastrointestinal problems include ischemic bowel and colitis; pulmonary complications include: nasal septum perforation, gingival ulceration, perennial rhinitis, sinusitis, hemoptysis, upper airway obstruction, fibrosis, hypersensitivity pneumonitis, epiglottitis, pulmonary hemorrhage, pulmonary hypertension, pulmonary edema, emphysema, interstitial fibrosis, and hypersensitivity pneumonia; neurologic complications: stroke, seizure, status epilepticus, headache, delirium, depression, hypersomnia, and cognitive defects; sleep issues include hypersomnia in withdrawal; perioperative effects consist of: hypersomnia and depression in withdrawal, inability to separate postoperative neurologic complications from drug effects, and complications due to underlying pulmonary disease; and musculoskeletal effects of rhabdomyolysis.

Inhalants

These include three classes of compounds: volatile alkyl nitrites, nitrous oxide, and volatile solvents/fuels/anesthetics. Deaths as a result of abuse are well known. Death results from behavioral toxicity and overdose. The solvents as a class produce significant intoxication and anesthetic effects at high concentrations. The usual scenario is loss of consciousness with overdose and lethal concentrations of the compounds. The proximate cause of death is CNS depression with respiratory arrest. There are also reports of acute cardiotoxicity with cardiac arrest. The major areas of effects are the brain, nose/mouth, lungs, liver, and kidneys. The classic neurotoxins are hexane and methyl-n-butylketone (MBK). These solvents produce axonopathies. Leaded gasoline causes demyelination. The inhalants show significant neuropathies with loss of white matter, brain atrophy, and damage to neural pathways. Coupled with these physiologic effects are the high rates of psychiatric disorders with inhalant abuse. One recent study found that 70 % of inhalant abusers met criteria for at least one lifetime mood, anxiety, or personality disorder, and 38 % had a mood disorder in the last year of study [16].

Chronic solvent abusers demonstrate irritation of the eyes, nose, and mouth with rhinitis, nose bleeds, conjunctivitis, and skin rash. Chronic use also leads to inflammation of the lungs with chronic cough. There may also be pulmonary edema, bronchospasm, bronchitis, granulomatosis, and even airway burns. The liver may be damaged particularly with the halogenated hydrocarbons like carbon tetrachloride. Glomerulonephritis and kidney stones have been reported and even acute tubular necrosis with toluene. Benzene and vinyl chloride are known carcinogens. Nitrites and methylene chloride can cause methemoglobinemia.

Prevention

No discussion of substance abuse would be complete without discussion of prevention. There are several excellent screening tools for initiating discussion of the risk for and prevention of substance abuse. One such tool is the "SBIRT" or "Screening, Brief Intervention, Referral to Treatment" tool. SBIRT is an all-encompassing, integrated means to assess for early intervention and treatment for individuals with substance abuse disorders, and those who are at risk for developing these disorders. The SBIRT may be utilized in primary care offices, ERs, trauma centers, public health clinics, and other healthcare settings to allow opportunity for early intervention for at-risk individuals before significant consequences.

Screening involves the quick assessment of the severity of the substance use and identifies appropriate levels of treatment.

Brief intervention provides emphasis on increasing insight and awareness about substance use and motivation for behavioral changes.

Referral to treatment provides those identified as needing more extensive treatment with access to specialty care.

Provider involvement is key to the success of the interventions. More complete information may be obtained at www.samhsa.gov/sbirt/resources (Accessed 10/30/2015).

Screening for alcohol abuse may be done with the simple "CAGE" questionnaire. Two "yes responses" indicate that there is a possibility of alcoholism and possible abuse investigated further. The questions are as follows:

1. Have you ever felt you needed to CUT down on your drinking?
2. Have people ANNOYED you by criticizing your drinking?
3. Have you ever felt GUILTY about drinking?
4. Have you ever felt you needed a drink first thing in the morning (EYE-opener) to steady your nerves or to get rid of a hangover?

Screening for drugs may be accomplished with the "Drug Abuse Screening Test-10" or DAST-10. This tool consists of ten questions to help score the level of drug abuse. The questions are (yes or no, and, refer to previous 12 months):

1. Have you used drugs other than those required for medical reasons?
2. Do you abuse more than one drug at a time?
3. Are you always able to stop using drugs when you want to? (If never used drugs, answer yes)
4. Have you had "blackouts" or "flashbacks" as a result of drug use?
5. Do you ever feel bad or guilty about your drug use? If never used drugs, choose "No".
6. Does your spouse (or parents) ever complain about your involvement with drugs?
7. Have you neglected your family because of your drug use?
8. Have you engaged in illegal activities in order to obtain drugs?
9. Have you ever experienced withdrawal symptoms (felt sick) when you stopped taking drugs?
10. Have you had medical problems as a result of your drug use (e.g., memory loss, hepatitis, convulsions, bleeding, etc)? (see https://www.drugabuse.gov/sites/default/files/DAST-10pdf)

Once these items have been scored, the interpretation involves how high the scoring of the questions answered is for the individual. The scoring is as follows:

DAST-10 score	Drug abuse	Suggested action
0	No problems reported	None at this time
1–2	Low level	Monitor, reassess
3–4	Moderate level	Further investigation
6–8	Substantial level	Intensive assessment
9–10	Severe level	Intensive assessment

The most important part of screening remains the initiation of frank conversation with our patients regarding substance and alcohol abuse. As screening becomes a part of routine care, it becomes more and more comfortable to the providers and the patients. Our patients will be grateful we cared enough to begin this serious and potentially life-saving discussion.

References

1. Dani JA, Harris RS. Nicotine addiction and comorbidity with alcohol abuse and mental illness. Nat Neurosci. 2005;11: 146–1470.
2. Mathers CD, Loncar D. Projections of global mortality and burden of disease from 2002 to 2030. PLoS Med. 2006;3(11), e442.
3. Benowitz NL. Clinical pharmacology of nicotine: implications for understanding, preventing, and treating tobacco addiction. Clin Pharmacol Ther. 2008;83(4):531–41.
4. Centers for Disease Control and Prevention. Vital signs: current cigarette smoking among adults aged ≥ 18 years with mental illness-United States, 2009-2001. MMWR Morb Wkly Rep. 2013;62(5):81–7.
5. CDC. Annual smoking attributable mortality, years of potential life lost, and economic costs: United States, 1995-1999. MMWR Morb Mortal Wkly Rep. 2001;51(14):300–3.

6. Benowitz NL. Basic cardiovascular research and its implications for the medicinal use of nicotine. J Am Coll Cardiol. 2003;4(3): 497–8.

7. Armentano P. Cannabis and psychomotor performance: a rational review of the evidence and implications for public policy. Drug Test Anal. 2013;5(1):52–6.

8. Bava S, Tapert SF. Adolescent brain development and the risk for alcohol and other drug problems. Neuropsychol Rev. 2010; 20:398–413.

9. Meieer MH, Caspi A, Ambler A, et al. Persistent cannabis users show neuropsychological decline form childhood to midlife. Proc Natl Acad Sci U S A. 2012;109(40):E2657–64.

10. SAMSA (Substance Abuse and Mental Health Services Administration). Drug abuse warning network: national estimates of drug-related emergency room visits. Rockville: Substance Abuse and Mental Health Services Administration; 2009.

11. Krantz MJ, Lewkowiez L, Hays H, et al. Torsades de pointes associated with very-high-dose methadone. Ann Intern Med. 2002;137:501–4.

12. O'Conner AD, Rusyniak DE, Bruno A. Cerebrovascular and cardiovascular complications of alcohol and sympathomimetic drug abuse. Med Clin North Am. 2005;89:1343–58.

13. Qureshi AI, Suri FK, Guterman LR, et al. Cocaine use and the likelihood of nonfatal myocardial infarction and stroke. Circulation. 2001;103:502–6.

14. Afonso L, Mohammad T, Thatai D. Crack whips the heart: a review of the cardiovascular toxicity of cocaine. Am J Cardiol. 2007;100:1040–3.

15. Wolff AJ, O'Donnell AE. Pulmonary effects of illicit drug use. Clin Chest Med. 2004;25:203–16.

16. Wu LT, Howard MO. Psychiatric disorders in inhalant users: result from the National Epidemiologic Survey on Alcohol and Related Conditions. Drug Alcohol Depend. 2007;88:146–55.

Chapter 6
Pregnancy Effects

Byron C. Calhoun

The national substance abuse rates have been estimated to be between 2.8 and 19 % [1–3]. The most recent data available (2013 data) reported by the Substance Abuse and Mental Health Services Administration (SAMHSA) in 2015 found a 2.6 % rate of illicit drug use in the United States in 2013 [4]. However, most concerning are the much higher rates of substance use in the reproductive age cohorts. The rates at 12–17 years of age were 3.5 %; the 18–25 years of age an astonishing 7.4 %; and the 26–44 years of age 3.1 %. This data demonstrates the significant public health issue substance abuse and illicit drug use in women's reproductive health particularly in obstetrical care. SAMHSA depends heavily on the use of survey data, self-reporting, and reporting from healthcare entities. The data are not generally linked to actual substance testing or necessarily verified with biologic samples.

In light of these findings, the American College of Obstetricians and Gynecologists (ACOG) and the American

B.C. Calhoun, MD, FACOG, FACS, FASAM, MBA (✉)
Department of Obstetrics and Gynecology, West Virginia
University-Charleston, Charleston, WV, USA
e-mail: Byron.calhoun@camc.org

© Springer International Publishing Switzerland 2016 101
B.C. Calhoun, T. Lewis (eds.), *Tobacco Cessation and
Substance Abuse Treatment in Women's Healthcare*,
DOI 10.1007/978-3-319-26710-4_6

Society of Addiction Medicine (ASAM) have both developed guidelines for recommendations related to drug use during pregnancy [5, 6]. The ACOG and ASAM guidelines are summarized below:

ACOG

- Universal screening for drug use in females of reproductive age.
- Screening at first prenatal or intake visit and at least once per trimester thereafter.
- Consider drug testing (with patient consent) when screening tests are positive.
- Refer for substance abuse treatment for all pregnant women who have evidence of drug use in pregnancy.
- Protect physician–patient relationship.

ASAM

- Prenatal education about all drugs for all pregnant patients.
- Universal screening to identify "at risk" women including repeat follow-up assessments.
- Culturally competent public prevention programs to educate the public about realistic dangers of drug use in pregnancy.
- Education of healthcare providers in the care and management of women with evidence of drug use before, during, and after pregnancy.
- Women who are pregnant should receive priority admission to substance treatment facilities.

Adolescents present a particularly vulnerable population and may need more detailed screening questions about alcohol and drug use with regard to driving, self-esteem, relaxation, interpersonal relations including family, and any type of trouble (school or legal). Adolescents also present issues in confidentiality that must be dealt with in the context of substance abuse. Consultation with various state guidelines and legislation is recommended.

Tobacco

Tobacco abuse continues to be a major problem among adolescents. SAMHSA 2015 (using 2013 data as last completed year of analysis) reported that 5.6 % of adolescents age 12–17 (approximately 1.4 million adolescents) admitted to using cigarettes within a month of the 2013 survey [7]. Cigarette usage was also higher in metropolitan areas (8.4 %) compared to rural areas (5.1 %). SAMHSA further reported that the number of US adolescents using cigarettes had dropped from 9.0 to 5.6 % from 2009 to 2013. There were significant drops in usage reported in whites, blacks, and Hispanics. Even so, these are concerning statistic given the fact these young women are in the reproductive age range and suffer the same ill-effects of tobacco on pregnancy.

Maternal cigarette smoking during pregnancy has always been a concern due to its association with poor maternal and fetal outcome. The association between maternal tobacco abuse and the elevated risk for low birth weight, preterm delivery, and IUGR are all well documented in the literature [8]. In 2002, 11.4 % of women giving birth in the United States admitted to smoking during their pregnancy [9]. Although this has improved from years past, in West Virginia the percentage of women smoking during pregnancy has increased to 35.7 %. From 2000 to 2005, West Virginia experienced an increase in smoking rates during all stages of reproduction: before, during, and after pregnancy [10].

Evidence regarding the negative effects of nicotine on fetal development is well established in existing literature. Tobacco use during pregnancy has been shown to cause significant changes within maternal and fetal cell transcriptomes involved in the deregulation of many biological processes critical for both growth and development [11]. It has also been found that tobacco use also causes significant reductions of placental vascularization [12]. These findings are related to subsequent fetal morbidities including small for gestational age infants (SGA), intrauterine growth retardation (IUGR), low birth weight, premature rupture of membranes, stillbirth, and sudden infant death syndrome [13–16]. In addition, smoking increases the risk for the following: cryptorchism in males [17], orofacial clefts [18], and asthma and bronchopulmonary hyperreactivity [19,20]. Perinatal morbidities include increased risk for placental abruption [21], fetal malpresentation [22], preterm birth [23, 24], and stillbirth [25, 26]. Mental disorders are also increased among women with nicotine dependence [27]. Recently findings about prenatal exposure to tobacco include an association of reduced brain growth in fetuses [28]; significant increase in attention deficit/hyperactivity, oppositional defiant disorder, and conduct disorder [29, 30]; and risk of poor school performance during adolescence [31].

England et al. 2013 demonstrated that preterm, premature rupture of membranes (PPROM) increased <28 by an odds ratio of 5.28 [CI 2.20–12.7]; <32 weeks odds ratio 2.36 [1.09–5.11]; <37 weeks odds ratio 1.97 (CI 1.32–2.94); and >37 weeks odds ratio [CI 0.92–11.0] with >10 cigarettes per day [32]. Kyrklund-Blomberg and Cnattingius 1998 found in a study of approximately 70,000 smokers in Sweden an almost double the rate of PPROM among nonsmokers (6.5/1000) versus smokers (11.5/1000) who smoked at least 10 cigarettes a day [33].

Baba et al. 2013 found an increased risk of stillbirth with an odds ratio of 1.59 (1.40–1.80) [34]. Varner et al. 2014 compared women who never smoked to those who reported smoking 1–9 cigarettes with an increased odds ratio of 1.77 (95 % CI 1.13–2.80) and for those smoking ≥10 cigarettes per day had an odds ratio for stillbirth of 2.17 (95 % CI 1.25–3.78) [35]. In another study by Hyland et al. 2013 demonstrated an increase in stillbirth rate with an odds ratio of 1.44 (1.20–1.73) in smokers [36]. These researchers also found that high levels of secondhand smoke (SHS) exposure, women with >10 years of childhood exposure, adult home >20 years, and adult work exposure >10 years had an adjusted odds ratio of 1.55 for stillbirth (95 % CI 1.21–1.97) [36]. They also found in this same cohort of high SHS exposure and adjusted odds ratio of 1.17 (95 % 1.05–1.30) and an adjusted odds ratio of 1.61 (95 % CI 1.16–2.24) for ectopic pregnancy [36].

The attribution of tobacco to IUGR in the United States has been stated as about 13.7 % of all births [37]. Horta et al.

1997 found an increased odds ratio for IUGR of 1.59 (95 % 1.30–1.95) in the cohort of patients who smoked compared to those who did not smoke [38]. They found a direct dose–response association with the number of cigarettes smoked and the risk of IUGR [38]. Therefore, since pregnant women who use tobacco are at an increased risk for adverse perinatal outcomes, their pregnancy is considered high-risk and requires monitoring and surveillance. This surveillance includes ultrasounds to monitor growth after 28–32 weeks, non-stress testing/biophysical profiles for fetal well-being beginning at 28–32 weeks, and/or, fetal Doppler surveillance. Most practitioners consider these patients significant high risk for adverse perinatal outcome and do not allow them to progress beyond 40 0/7 weeks gestation. Many suggest induction of labor at 39 0/7 weeks gestation with a favorable cervix ought to be considered in tobacco abuse patients due to their high-risk status.

Opioids

Substance abuse in pregnancy has well-known deleterious effects on neonates. These effects differ with respect to the substance ingested and can include neonatal abstinence syndrome (NAS), low birth weight, intrauterine fetal demise, and structural abnormalities such as gastroschisis.

The national substance abuse rates have been estimated to be between 2.8 and 19 % [1–3]. These reported rates vary based upon the population screened and the method of screening used. The lowest number reported in the study by Ebrahim and Gfroerer utilized a population survey of the entire United States [1] while the highest rates reported (19 %) by Azadi and Dildy utilized urine toxicology testing [3]. Chasnoff et al. developed a self-reporting screening tool that estimated that 15 % of the population studied continued to use substances of abuse after becoming aware of the pregnancy [2].

Opioid dependence, including methadone maintenance, has been linked to fetal death, growth restriction, preterm birth, meconium aspiration, and NAS [39, 40]. NAS may be present in 60–90 % of neonates exposed in utero with up to 70 % of affected neonates with central nervous system (CNS) irritability that may progress to seizures [40]. Up to 50 % of neonates may experience respiratory issues, feeding problems, and failure to thrive [41]. These issues are present as well in those infants whose mothers' are on methadone maintenance [42]. However, with methadone the onset of NAS may be delayed for several weeks [42]. Some authors recommend 5–8 days of maternal hospitalization while their neonates' undergo observation for NAS [43]. However, most insurance plans will not reimburse for the prolonged uncomplicated maternal stay while awaiting neonatal detoxification.

A randomized controlled study of 175 pregnant patients (89 methadone/86 buprenorphine) comparing methadone to buprenorphine by Jones et al. 2010 found both methadone and buprenorphine found that 57 % (41/75) of neonates had NAS with methadone and 47 % (27/58) of neonates had NAS with buprenorphine [42]. The buprenorphine cohort had shorter hospital stays (10.0 versus 17.5 days, $P < 0.0091$) and shorter days of treatment for NAS (4.1 versus 9.9 days, $P < 0.003125$) [44].

The incidence of opioid relapse in pregnant opioid abusing women is very high with 41–96 % relapsing. This mirrors the relapse rate of the general population at 1 month of 65–80 % [45, 46]. Over 90 % of patients will relapse at 6 months after medication-assisted withdrawal [47]. Buprenorphine (Subutex™) appears to have no difference in outcomes with regard to treatment of opiate addicted women. The same NAS and neonatal affects are present [48].

Recent work published by Montgomery et al. 2006 compared the performance of meconium samples versus the testing of umbilical cord tissue [49]. This study showed concordance of the testing methods that correlated at or above 90 % for all substances analyzed. Follow-up work included a study in which umbilical cord samples were collected and tested if high-risk criteria for substance abuse were identified. Out of this cohort, 157 of 498 (32 %) cords tested positive for substances of abuse [50]. Stitely et al. 2010 found similar results in their study of cord samples in eight regional hospitals in West Virginia with 146/759 (19.2 %) of umbilical cord samples collected at delivery that were positive for either illicit substances or alcohol [51].

The number of newborns treated for NAS has increased dramatically in West Virginia. In data collected from the Cabell Huntington Hospital in Huntington, WV, the number of neonates treated for NAS increased from 25 in 2003 to 70 in 2007 [51]. The cost difference in the care of an otherwise healthy neonate with NAS compared to a normal full-term healthy neonate was estimated to be $3934 in the Cabell-Huntington cohort. Because of the added costs associated with the increased risk of prematurity, the average cost of all infants with NAS was $36,000 compared to $2000 for a normal neonate [52].

Unfortunately, according to SAMHSA 2015 (using 2013 data as last completed year of analysis), over 6.9 million people age 12 years or older had illicit drug dependence or abuse [53]. Further, SAMHSA reports the dismal statistic that only 13.4 % (about some 917,000 treated/6.9 million people with a problem) received treatment. Most startling as well was that 8 out of 10 people with illicit drug dependence or abuse did not perceive a need for treatment for their illicit drug use. Considerable disconnect exists between people's perceptions of illicit drug use with addiction and the reality of addiction their lives. It is not clear from the SAMHSA data that treatment is not always available with a lack of services for addictions and mental health or that the individuals have never been questioned or confronted regarding their illicit substance abuse or addiction. Better treatment is needed not only for pregnant women but all drug-dependent individuals. Much work remains in this realm.

Cocaine, Amphetamines, and Stimulants

Cocaine has known adverse effects in pregnancy. In particular, it has been linked with placenta-associated syndromes (PAS). PAS include placental abruption, oligohydramnios, placental infarction, gestational hypertension, preeclampsia, and eclampsia. Mbah et al. 2012 found that cocaine increased the risk for PAS by 58 % and noted an increased OR of 1.48 (95 % CI 1.33–1.66) [54]. They also found the most increased risk with cocaine exposure in placental abruption with an OR of 2.79 (95 % CI 2.19–3.55).

Exposure to cocaine prenatally investigated by Bauer et al. 2005 found several clinical and physical findings including: born 1 week earlier, weighing 322 g less, 1.7 cm shorter, and 1.0 cm smaller head circumference [55]. Exposed infants also had a significantly higher frequency of CNS symptoms with OR of 1.7 (99 % CI 1.2–2.2), autonomic nervous system symptoms with OR 1.5 (99 % CI 1.0–2.1), and increased infection rates with OR 3.1 (99 % CI 1.8–5.4). Opiates plus cocaine had an additive effect for CNS/ANS signs with an OR of 4.8 (95 % CI 2.9–7.9). Tobacco plus cocaine was also additive with an OR of 1.3 (CI 95 % 1.04–1.55) with ½ppd and OR of 1.4 (95 % CI 1.2–2.6) with 1 ppd. Cocaine exposure also increased the risk of IUGR, prematurity, and low birth weight with an OR of 2.24 for IUGR, 1.25 for prematurity, and 3.59 for low birth weight [56].

Neurobehavior deviations in children exposed to cocaine have been found to be increased in the motor, sensory, and integrative functions. These neurologic "soft-signs" include ten different areas: speech, balance, coordination, double simultaneous stimulation (extinction), gait, sequential finger-thumb opposition, muscle tone, graphesthesia (inability to identify forms with tactile stimulation, i.e., a number drawn in palm), stereognosis (inability to identify an object by touch), and choreiform signs [57]. Cocaine was also associated by Breslau et al. 1999, with subnormal IQ and learning disorders with children with normal IQs [58]. These effects were found to be present particularly in the behavioral issues in longitudinal studies of children from birth 7 years of age [59]. These effects even after controlling for substance use, demographic factors, family violence, and family members psychological issues. Lester et al. 2003 even estimated that the cost to society with regard to special needs and education cost over $25,000,000 a year for cocaine exposure [60].

Amphetamine abuse, like cocaine, has been associated in pregnancy with vaginal bleeding, abruption placenta, placenta previa, premature rupture of membranes, decreased head circumference, low birth weight, tremulousness, irritability, poor feeding, and autonomic instability [61]. Nguyen et al. 2010 found a significant risk for SGA infants when adjusting for covariates of alcohol, tobacco, and marijuana use [62]. The increased OR was 2.05 compared to non-amphetamine abusers (95 % CI 1.24–3.37).

Treatment of amphetamine abuse with fluoxetine and imipramine may be useful but is not a panacea for treatment. A recent review by the *Cochrane Collaboration* in 2001 (reissued in 2009) noted that medications are of limited use in treatment of amphetamine abuse [63]. They note that there are very limited trials at this time to be able to suggest what is the best way to treat amphetamine abuse.

Alcohol

Heavy use of alcohol is a known teratogen leading to fetal alcohol syndrome (FAS) which includes CNS dysfunction, microcephaly, learning disabilities, and facial abnormalities. Affected individuals may have some or all of the manifestations of the syndrome.

Fetal alcohol syndrome (FAS) includes the following classic phenotype and includes:

- Evidence of growth retardation (prenatal or postnatal): height and weight equal to or less than the tenth percentile, corrected for racial norms and sex.
- Evidence of deficient brain growth and/or abnormal morphogenesis, including one or more of the following: structural brain anomalies or head circumference equal to or less than the tenth percentile (microcephaly).
- Evidence of a characteristic pattern of minor facial anomalies, including two or more of the following: short palpebral fissures (equal to or less than the tenth percentile), thin vermillion border of upper lip, and smooth philtrum.

Fetal alcohol spectrum disorders include the following:

- FAS with and without confirmed maternal alcohol exposure.
- Partial FAS: This is a diagnostic classification that includes known or unknown maternal alcohol exposure. It includes minor facial anomalies and evidence of other either prenatal and/or postnatal growth delay or structural brain abnormalities or microcephaly.
- Alcohol related birth defects (ARBD): Due to exposure to alcohol and may cause structural defects in multiple organ systems. This includes anomalies in cardiac (atrial-septal defect, ventriculoseptal defect, conotruncal anomalies), skeletal (radioulnar synostosis and vertebral defects), renal (aplastic/hypoplastic/dysplastic kidneys), eyes (strabismus, ptosis, vascular and nerve anomalies), and ears (conductive and sensorineural hearing defects). There may also be minor anomalies of the hands, ears, and chest wall with pectus carinatum/excavatum.
- Alcohol related neurodevelopmental disorder (ARND) which includes significant cognitive and behavioral abnormalities. There is a marked loss of complex task completion, higher level receptive language, expressive language disorder, and even disordered behaviors.

Shankaran et al. 2007 found that neurobehavioral deviations in children exposed to cocaine and have been found to be increased in the motor, sensory, and integrative functions [64]. These neurologic "soft-signs" include ten different areas: speech, balance, coordination, double simultaneous stimulation (extinction), gait, sequential finger-thumb opposition, muscle tone, graphesthesia (inability to identify forms with tactile stimulation, i.e., a number drawn in palm), stereognosis (inability to identify an object by touch), and choreiform signs. Children exposed to both cocaine and alcohol had an increased OR of 6.4 (95 % CI 2.5–16.6) of having a two or more of the soft signs of abnormal behaviors compared to unexposed children [64]. Children exposed in utero to binge drinking also had increased OR of 3.6 (95 % CI 1.0–12.8) of having at least two abnormal neurobehavioral findings [64].

The prevalence of FAS and FASD varies across various populations but there are affected adults and children in all races and ethnic groups. In the USA, the estimate of the alcohol use disorders is estimated at 0.5–2 per 1000 live births with FAS. FASD appears to be more common and is estimated that up to 1 % of live births affected [65].

These neurologic deficits will persist into adulthood. No safe amount of alcohol ingestion has been found in pregnancy and there is no treatment for the effects of alcohol on the fetus. Total abstinence is recommended in pregnancy. Unfortunately, alcohol rehabilitation has had little written in pregnancy and until recently no ability to verify chronic use of alcohol due to its volatile nature and inability to test for its presence.

Lastly, treatment for alcohol dependence or abuse, according to the SAMHSA 2013 data, appears no better than that for substance dependence or abuse. SAMHSA reports some 17.3 million people greater than age 12 years have been found to have alcohol dependence or abuse [66]. Of that 17.3 million, only 1.1 million (6.3 %) received treatment. Nine out of ten individuals with alcohol dependence or abuse did not perceive a need for treatment for their alcohol use. There was no difference in treatment rates by health insurance status, socioeconomic status, or rural versus urban areas. Once again, perceptions by individuals is sorely lacking regarding the harmful effects of their alcohol dependence or abuse. Also, it is not possible from the SAMHSA data to determine if treatment is not available due to a lack of services for addictions and mental health, or, that the individuals have never been questioned or confronted regarding their illicit substance abuse or addiction.

Sedatives

Barbiturates appear to be part of the anticonvulsant drug syndrome consisting of an increase in major malformations, growth retardation, and hypoplasia of the midface and fingers. The relative risk for major malformations with anticonvulsant therapy was found to be 4.2 [67]. Also, the use of high dose barbiturates at term may lead to respiratory depression and withdrawal in the neonate.

Benzodiazepine use has been associated with possible cleft lip and palate but the data appear inconclusive due to exposure to other substances, particularly alcohol. Abuse of the benzodiazepines near delivery may result in a neonate with poor muscle tone and respiratory depression.

Sedative withdrawal is less common than with the opioids and may be delayed with long acting benzodiazepines such as diazepam. Most neonates do not require therapy but for severe withdrawal Phenobarbital is the drug of choice. The dosing generally begins orally or intramuscularly at 2–4 mg/kg of body weight every 8 h. The dose is then tapered 10–20 % per day over 5–10 days [68]. Benzodiazepine dependence and detoxification must be done gradually to reduce symptoms. Little has been written about benzodiazepine detoxification in pregnancy.

Inhalants/Solvents

Inhalants and solvents represent a small and select group of pregnant patients. Estimates note that up to 12,000 women may use inhalants while pregnant [69]. There is a suggestion of decreased fertility and spontaneous abortion with inhalants [69]. It is not clear if the infertility is a direct effect of the inhalants on ovarian and testicular function or a secondary effect due to CNS effects on the hypothalamic axis. Clinical reports note that the adverse effects of solvents on the fetus include low birth weight, facial and other physical abnormalities, microcephaly, and delayed neurologic/physiologic maturation.

Marijuana

Marijuana remains the most frequently used illicit drug in the Western countries with roughly 20 million (7.5 %) of adult population using marijuana in last month [70]. Prevalence of use in pregnancy ranges from 3 to 34 % in the literature [71]. It is estimated that up to one third of the active psychogenic compound of delta-9-tetrahydrocannabinol (THC) crosses the placenta to the fetus with smoking marijuana [72]. Studies report increased rates of fetal distress, growth retardation, and adverse neurodevelopmental outcomes with prenatal exposure to cannabis. Also, several studies note that infants born to regular cannabis users have increased tremors, exaggerated startle response, and poor habituation to novel stimuli [73]. This pathogenic impact is further substantiated with epidemiological and clinical studies documenting impulsive behavior, social deficit, cognitive impairment, consumption of addictive substances, and psychiatric disorders with in utero exposure. The studies found that by age 10 years, marijuana exposed children in particular have increased hyperactivity, inattention, and impulsive behaviors. These children also have increased delinquency and externalizing behavioral problems compared to age comparable children without exposure to THC [74]. A recent case control study by Varner et al. found that THC use increased the rate of stillbirth with an OR of 2.3 (95 % CI 1.13–4.81) [35]. The effects of marijuana on preterm birth have been mixed but at least two large Australian retrospective studies demonstrate a possible increased risk of preterm birth. These two studies found an increased OR of 1.5 (CI 95 % 1.1–1.9) in one study and preterm birth rate of 18.8 % versus 5.8 % ($P < 0.001$) in the other [75, 76]. There does not appear to be evidence at this time in the literature that marijuana use is associated either decreased birth weight or congenital anomalies. There is evidence to support a mild withdrawal syndrome similar to opioid withdrawal associated with cannabis exposure. Therapy is rarely indicated.

Comorbidities

Comorbidities with multiple psychiatric issues in the patients with substance abuse issues must be considered. The 2011 USA National Survey on Drug Use and Health found that

17.5 % of adults with a mental illness had a co-occurring substance use disorder; involving some 7.98 million people [77]. Significant numbers of patients with substance dependence have affective disorders including: depression, mania, schizoaffective disorders, schizophrenia, borderline personality, and bipolar disorders. A study by Kessler et al, 1994 in the United States, attempting to assess the prevalence of dual diagnosis with substance abuse and mental illness, found that 47 % of patients with schizophrenia had a substance misuse disorder at some time in their life [78], and Regier et al. 1990 found the chances of developing a substance abuse disorder were significantly higher among patients suffering from a psychotic illness than in the those without a psychotic illness [79]. Another study looked at the extent of substance abuse in a group of 187 chronically mentally ill patients living in a community setting. According to the clinician's evaluations, about 33 % of the sample used alcohol, street drugs, or both, during the 6 months before evaluation [80].

Therefore, many authors recently note that detoxification must be linked with a combination of behavioral therapy with contingency management therapy [81, 82]. Behavioral therapy consists of the use of addictions counselors and counseling to assist substance and alcohol abusers to remain drug and alcohol free. Finally, many agree the liberal use of biologic testing for abstinence verification should be a part of any robust addictions programs. Monitoring of compliance assists in building accountability in the patients and demonstrates commitment to consistent oversight in achieving sobriety and health in the individuals.

References

1. Ebrahim SH, Gfroerer J. Pregnancy-related substance use in the United States during 1996-1998. Obstet Gynecol. 2003; 101(2):374–9.
2. Chasnoff IJ, McGourty RF, Bailey GW, Hutchins E, Lightfoot SO, Pawson LL, Fahey C, May B, Brodie P, McCulley L, Campbell J. The 4P's Plus screen for substance use in pregnancy: clinical application and outcomes. J Perinatol. 2005;25(6):368–74.

3. Azadi A, Dildy III GA. Universal screening for substance abuse at the time of parturition. Am J Obstet Gynecol. 2008;198(5):e30–2. Epub 2008 Feb 14.
4. Substance Abuse and Mental Health Services Administration. Behavioral Health Barometer: United States, 2014. HHS Publication No. SMA-15-4895. Rockville: Substance Abuse and Mental Health Services Administration; 2015. p. 14.
5. American College of Obstetricians and Gynecologist Committee on Health Care for Underserved Women and the American Society of Addiction Medicine. ACOG Committee Opinion #524: opioid abuse, dependence, and addiction in pregnancy.
6. American Society of Addiction Medicine. Public policy statement on women, alcohol, and other drugs, and pregnancy. Chevy Chase: American Society of Addiction Medicine; 2011.
7. Substance Abuse and Mental Health Services Administration. Behavioral Health Barometer: United States, 2014. HHS Publication No. SMA-15-4895. Rockville: Substance Abuse and Mental Health Services Administration; 2015. p. 4.
8. Kalinka J, Hanke W, Sobala W. Impact of prenatal tobacco smoke exposure, as measured by midgestation serum cotinine levels, on fetal biometry and umbilical flow velocity waveforms. Am J Perinatol. 2005;22(1):41–7.
9. Centers for Disease Control and Prevention. Smoking during pregnancy — United States, 1990-1992. MMWR. 2004;53:911–5.
10. Tong VT, Jones JR, Dietz PM, D'Angelo D, Bombard JM. Trends in smoking before, during, and after pregnancy — pregnancy risk assessment monitoring system (pRAMS), United States, 31 sites, 2000-2005. MMWR Surveill Summ. 2009;58:1–31.
11. Votavova H, Dostalova MM, Fejglova K, Vasikova A, Krejcik Z, Pastorkova A, Tabashidze N, Topinka J, Veleminsky Jr M, Sram RJ, Brdicka R. Transcriptome alteration in maternal and fetal cells induced by tobacco smoke. Placenta. 2011;32(10):763–70.
12. Ortigosa S, Friguls B, Joya X, Martinez S, Marinoso ML, Alameda F, Vall O, Garcia-Algar O. Feto-placental morphological effects of prenatal exposure to drugs of abuse. Reprod Toxicol. 2012;34(1):73–9.
13. Jaddoe VWV, Verburg BO, de Ridder MAJ, Hofman A, Mackenbach JP, Moll HA, Steegers EAP, Witteman JCM, et al. Maternal smoking and fetal growth characteristics in different periods of pregnancy. The generation R study. Am J Epidemiol. 2007;165:1207–15.
14. Ingvarsson RF, Bjarnason AO, Dagbjarsson A, Hardardottir H, Haraldsson A, Thorkelsson T, et al. The effects of smoking in

pregnancy on factors influencing fetal growth. Acta Paediatr. 2007;96:383–6.

15. Okah FA, Hoff GL, Dew P, Cai J, et al. Cumulative and residual risks of small for gestational age neonates after changing pregnancy-smoking related behaviors. Am J Perinatol. 2007;24:191–6.

16. Villalbi JR, Salvador J, Cano-Serral G, Rodriguez-Sanz MC, Borrell C. Maternal smoking, social class and outcomes of pregnancy. Paediatr Perinat Epidemiol. 2007;21:441–7.

17. Jensen MS, Toft G, Thulstrup AM, Bonde JP, Olsen J, et al. Cryptorchidism according to maternal gestational smoking. Epidemiology. 2007;19(2):220–5.

18. Honein MA, Rasmussen SA, Reefhuis J, Romitti PA, Lammer EJ, Sun L, Correa A, et al. Maternal smoking and environmental tobacco smoke exposure and the risk of orofacial clefts. Epidemiology. 2007;18(2):226–33.

19. Goksor E, Amark M, Alm B, Gustafsson PM, Wennergren G, et al. The impact of pre- and post-natal smoke exposure on future asthma and bronchial hyper-responsiveness. Acta Paediatr. 2007;96:1030–5.

20. Noakes PS, Thomas R, Lane C, Mori TA, Barden AE, Devadason SG, Prescott SL, et al. Association of maternal smoking with increased infant oxidative stress at 3 months of age. Thorax. 2007;62:714–7.

21. Ananth CV, Cnattingius S, et al. Influence of maternal smoking on placental abruption in successive pregnancies: a population-based prospective cohort study in Sweden. Am J Epidemiol. 2007;166:289–95.

22. Talas BB, Altinkaya SO, Talas H, Danisman N, Gungor T. Predictive factors and short-term fetal outcomes of breech presentation: a case-control study. Taiwan J Obstet Gynecol. 2008;47(4):402–7.

23. Andres RL, Day MC. Perinatal complications associated with maternal tobacco use. Semin Neonatal. 2000;5:231–41.

24. Cnattingius S. The epidemiology of smoking during pregnancy; smoking prevalence, maternal characteristics, and pregnancy outcomes. Nicotine Tob Res. 2004;6:125–40.

25. Hogberg L, Cnattingius S, et al. The influence of maternal smoking habits on the risk of subsequent stillbirth: is there a causal relation? BJOG. 2007;114:699–704.

26. Meeker JD, Missmer SA, Vitonis AF, Cramer DW, Hauser R, et al. Risk of spontaneous abortion in women with childhood exposure to parental cigarette smoke. Am J Epidemiol. 2007;156(5):571–5.

27. Goodwin RD, Keyes K, Simuro N, et al. Mental disorders and nicotine dependence among pregnant women in the United States. Obstet Gynecol. 2007;109:875–83.
28. Indredavik MS, Brubakk A, Romundstad P, Vik T, et al. Prenatal smoking exposure and psychiatric symptoms in adolescence. Acta Paediatr. 2007;96:377–82.
29. Nigg JT, Breslau N, et al. Prenatal smoking exposure, low birth weight, and disruptive behavior disorders. J Am Acad Child Adolesc Psychiatry. 2007;46(3):362–9.
30. Roza SJ, Verburg BO, Jaddoe VWV, Hofman A, Mackenbach JP, Steegers EAP, et al. Effects of maternal smoking in pregnancy on prenatal brain development. The general R study. Eur J Neurosci. 2007;25:611–7.
31. Lambe M, Hultman C, Torrang A, Maccabe J, Cnattingius S. Maternal smoking during pregnancy and school performance at age 16. Epidemiology. 2006;17:524–30.
32. England MC, Benjamin A, Abenhaim HA. Increased risk of preterm premature rupture of membranes at early gestational ages among maternal cigarette smokers. Am J Perinatal. 2013;30(10):821–6.
33. Kyrklund-Blomberg NB, Cnattingius S. Preterm birth and maternal smoking: risks related to gestational age and onset of delivery. Am J Obstet Gynecol. 1998;179:1051–5.
34. Baba S, Wikstrom AK, Stephanson O, Cnattingius S. Influence of snuff and smoking habits in early pregnancy on risks for stillbirth and early neonatal mortality. Nicotine Tob Res. 2014;16(1):78–83.
35. Varner MW, Silver RM, Rowland-Hogue CJ, et al. Association between stillbirth and illicit drug use and smoking during pregnancy. Obstet Gynecol. 2014;123(1):113–25.
36. Hyland A, Piazza KM, Hovey KM, Ockene JK, Andrews CA, RIvard C, Wactawski-Wende J. Association of lifetime active and passive smoking with spontaneous abortion, stillbirth, and tubal ectopic pregnancy: a cross-sectional analysis of historical data from the Women's Health Initiative. Tob Control. 2015;24(4):328–35.
37. Baba HS, Das A, Bauer CR, et al. Low birthweight and preterm births: etiologic fraction attributable to prenatal drug exposure. J Perinatol. 2005;25(10):631–7.
38. Horta BL, Victora CG, Menezes AM, Halpern R, Barros FC. Low birthweight, preterm births and intrauterine growth retardation in relation to maternal smoking. Paediatr Perinat Epidemiol. 1997;11(2):140–51.

39. Rementeria JL, Nunag NN. Narcotic withdrawal in pregnancy. Am J Obstet Gynecol. 1973;116:1152–6.
40. Hoegerman G, Schnoll SH. Methadone maintenance and withdrawal in pregnant opioid addicts. Clin Perinatol. 1991;18:51–76.
41. Briggs GG, Freeman RK, Yaffee SJ. Drugs in pregnancy and lactation. Baltimore: Williams and Wilkins; 1994. p. 557–8.
42. Cooper JR, Altman F, Brown BS, Czechowicz D, editors. Research on the treatment of narcotic addiction: State of the art. (NIDA Research Monograph 83-1201). Rockville: US Department of Health and Human Services; 1983.
43. Andres RL, Jones KL. Social and illicit drug use in pregnancy. In: Creasy RK, Resnick R, editors. Maternal-fetal medicine. Philadelphia: Saunders; 1994. p. 191–2.
44. Jones HE, Kaltenback K, Heil SH, Stine SM, Coyle MG, Arria AM, O'Grady KE, Selby P, Martin PR, Fischer G. Neonatal abstinence syndrome after methadone or buprenorphine exposure. N Engl J Med. 2010;363:2320–31.
45. Winklbaur B, Kopf N, Ebner N, Jung E, Thau K, Fischer G. Treating pregnant women dependent on opioids is not the same as treating pregnancy and opioid dependence: a knowledge synthesis for better treatment for women and neonates. Addiction. 2008;103:1429–40.
46. Chutuape MA, Jasinski DR, Fingerhood MI, Stitzer ML. One, three, and six month outcomes following brief inpatient opioid detoxification. Am J Drug Alcohol Abuse. 2001;27:19–44.
47. Gossop M, Green L, Phillips G, Bradley B. Lapse, relapse, and survival among opiate addicts immediately after treatment: a prospective follow-up study. Br J Psychiatry. 1989;154:348–53.
48. Jones HE, Johnson RE, Jasinski DR, O'Grady KE, Chisholm CA, Choo RE, Crocetti M, Dudas R, Harrow C, Huestis MA, Jansson LM, Lantz M, Lester BM, Milio L. Buprenorphine versus methadone in the treatment of pregnant opioid-dependent patients: effects on the neonatal abstinence syndrome. Drug Alcohol Depend. 2004;79:1–10.
49. Montgomery D, Plate C, Alder SC, Jones M, Jones J, Christensen RD. Testing for fetal exposure to illicit drugs using umbilical cord tissue vs meconium. J Perinatol. 2006;26(1):11–4.
50. Montgomery DP, Plate CA, Jones M, Jones J, Rios R, Lambert DK, Schumtz N, Wiedmeier SE, Burnett J, Ail S, Brandel D, Maichuck G, Durham CA, Henry E, Christensen RD. Using umbilical cord tissue to detect fetal exposure to illicit drugs: a multicentered study in Utah and New Jersey. J Perinatol. 2008;28(11):750–3. Epub 2008 Jul 3.

51. Stitely ML, Calhoun BC, Maxwell S, Nerhood R, Chaffin D. Prevalence of drug use in pregnant West Virginia patients. W V Med J. 2010;105:48–52.

52. Baxter FR, Nerhood R, Chaffin D. Characterization of babies discharged from Cabell Huntington Hospital during the calendar year 2005 with the diagnoses of neonatal abstinence syndrome. W V Med J. 2009;105(2):16–21.

53. Substance Abuse and Mental Health Services Administration. Behavioral Health Barometer: United States, 2014. HHS Publication No. SMA-15-4895. Rockville: Substance Abuse and Mental Health Services Administration; 2015. p. 19.

54. Mbah AK, Alio AP, Fombo DW, Bruder K, Dagne G, Salihu HM. Association between cocaine abuse in pregnancy and placenta-associated syndromes using propensity score matching approach. Early Hum Dev. 2012;88:333–7.

55. Bauer CR, Langer JC, Shankaran S, Bada HS, Wright LL, et al. Acute neonatal effects of cocaine exposure during pregnancy. Arch Pediatr Adolesc Med. 2005;159:824–34.

56. Bada HS, Das A, Bauer CR, Shankaran S, Lester B, Gard CC, et al. Low birth weight and preterm births: etiologies fraction attributable to prenatal drug exposure. J Perinatol. 2005;25:631–67.

57. Hertzig ME. Neurological "soft" signs in low-birthweight. Dev Med Child Neurol. 1981;23:778–91.

58. Breslau N, Chilcoat HD, Johnson EO, Andreski P, Lucia VC. Neurologic soft signs and low birth-weight: their association and neuropsychiatric implications. Biol Psychiatry. 2000;47:71–9.

59. Bada H, Das A, Bauer CR, Chankaran S, Lester B, LaGasse L, Hammond J, Wright LL, Higgins R. Impact of prenatal cocaine exposure on child behavior problems through school age. Pediatrics. 2007;119(2):e348–59.

60. Lester BM, Das A, LaGasse LL, Seifer R, Bauer CR, Shankaran S, et al. Prenatal cocaine exposure and 7-year outcome: IQ and special education. Pediatr Res. 2003;53:534A.

61. Phupong V, Darojn D. Amphetamine abuse in pregnancy: the impact on obstetric outcome. Arch Gynecol Obstet. 2007;276:167–70.

62. Nguyen D, Smith LM, LaGasse LL, Derauf C, Grant P, Shah R, Aria A, Huestis MA, Haning W, Strauss A, Grotta SD, Liu J, Lester BM. Intrauterine growth of infants exposed to prenatal methamphetamine: results from the Infant Development Environment and Lifestyle (IDEAL) Study. J Pediatr. 2010;157(2):337–9.

63. Srisurapanont M, Jarusuraisin N, Kittirattanapaiboon P. Treatment for amphetamine dependence and abuse. Cochrane Database Syst Rev. 2001;(4):CD003022.
64. Shankaran S, Lesster BM, Das A, Bauer CR, Bada HS, Lagasse L, Higgins R. Impact of maternal substance use during pregnancy on childhood outcome. Semin Fetal Neonatal Med. 2007;12(2): 143–50.
65. Sampson PD, Streissguth AP, Boostein FL, et al. Incidence of fetal alcohol syndrome and prevalence of alcohol-related neurodevelopmental disorder. Teratology. 1997;56:317–26.
66. Substance Abuse and Mental Health Services Administration. Behavioral Health Barometer: United States, 2014. HHS Publication No. SMA-15-4895. Rockville: Substance Abuse and Mental Health Services Administration; 2015. p. 17.
67. Holmes LB, Wyszinski DF, Lieberman E. The AED Pregnancy Registry: a 6 year experience. Arch Neurol. 2004;61:673–8.
68. Hudak ML, Tan RC. The Committee on Drugs, and the Committee on Fetus and Newborn. Neonatal Drug withdrawal. Pediatrics. 2012;129:e540–60.
69. Jones HE, Balster RL. Inhalant abuse in pregnancy. Obstet Gynecol Clin North Am. 1998;25:153–67.
70. Substance Abuse and Mental Health Services Administration. Results from the 2013 National Survey on Drug Use and Health: summary of national findings. www.samhsa.gov/data/sites/default/files/NSSATS2013Dir_CD.
71. National Institute on Drug Use. Nationwide trends. www.drugabuse.gov/publications/drugfacts/nationwide-trends.
72. Hurd Y, Wang X, Anderson V, Beck O, Minkoff H, Dow-Edwards D. Marijuana impairs growth in mid-gestation fetuses. Neurotoxicol Teratol. 2005;27:221–9.
73. Fried PA, Watkinson B, Dillon RF, Dulberg CS. Neonatal neurological status in a low-risk population after prenatal exposure to cigarettes, marijuana, and alcohol. J Dev Behav Pediatr. 1987;8:318–26.
74. Goldschmidt L, Day NL, Richardson GA. Effects of prenatal marijuana exposure on child behavior problems at age 10. Neurotoxicol Teratol. 2000;22:325–36.
75. Hyatbakhsh MR, Flenady VJ, Gibbons KS, et al. Birth outcomes associated with cannabis use before and during pregnancy. Pediatr Res. 2012;71:215–9.
76. Burns L, Mattick RP, Cooke M. The use of record linkage to examine illicit drug use in pregnancy. Addiction. 2006;101:873–82.

77. Substance Abuse and Mental Health Services Administration. Results from the 2011 National Survey on Drug Use and Health: mental health findings. Rockville: Substance Abuse and Mental Health Services Administration; 2012.
78. Kessler RC, McGonagle KA, Zhao S, Nelson CB, Hughes M, Eshleman S, Wittchen HU, Kendler KS. Lifetime and 12-month prevalence of DSM-III-R psychiatric disorders in the United States. Results from the National Comorbidity Survey. Arch Gen Psychiatry. 1994;51(1):8–19. doi:10.1001/archpsyc.51.1.8.
79. Regier DA, Farmer ME, Rae DS, Locke BZ, Keith SJ, Judd LL, Goodwin FK. Comorbidity of mental disorders with alcohol and other drug abuse. Results from the Epidemiologic Catchment Area (ECA) Study. JAMA. 1990;264(19):2511–8. doi:10.1001/jama.264.19.2511.
80. Drake RE, Wallach MA. Moderate drinking among people with severe mental illness. Hosp Community Psychiatry. 1993;44(8):780–2.
81. Dutra L, Statthopoulou G, Basden SL, Leyro TM, Powers MB, Otto MW. A meta-analytic review of psychosocial interventions for substance use disorders. Am J Psychiatry. 2008;165:179–87.
82. Moran P, Madgula RM, Gilvarry E, Findlay M. Substance misuse during pregnancy: its effects and treatment. Fetal Maternal Med Rev. 2009;20:1–16.

Chapter 7
Tobacco Cessation

Byron C. Calhoun

Background

West Virginia leads the nation in the percentage of women who smoke while pregnant (35.7 %) [1]. From 2000 to 2005, while most of the country experienced declines in smoking rates among pregnant women, West Virginia experienced an increase in smoking rates in all stages of reproduction. Smoking rates increased (36.2–45.8 %) prior to pregnancy, (29.4–35.7 %) during pregnancy, and (1.6–39.3 %) postpartum [1]. Findings from the West Virginia Bureau for Public Health, Health Statistics Center indicated that during 2005, pregnant women in West Virginia who smoked were 63.2 % more likely than nonsmoking pregnant women to have their child die during his/her first year of life. In addition, they were 97.4 % more likely to give birth to a low birth weight baby and 281.8 % more likely to have a child die from Sudden Infant Death Syndrome within his/her first year when compared to those who did not smoke.

Tobacco abuse continues to be a major problem among adolescents. SAMHSA 2015 (using 2013 data as last completed

B.C. Calhoun, MD, FACOG, FACS, FASAM, MBA (✉)
Department of Obstetrics and Gynecology, West Virginia
University-Charleston, Charleston, WV, USA
e-mail: Byron.calhoun@camc.org

© Springer International Publishing Switzerland 2016   123
B.C. Calhoun, T. Lewis (eds.), *Tobacco Cessation and
Substance Abuse Treatment in Women's Healthcare*,
DOI 10.1007/978-3-319-26710-4_7

year of analysis) reported that 5.6 % of adolescents age 12–17 (approximately 1.4 million adolescents) admitted to using cigarettes within a month of the 2013 survey [2]. Cigarette usage was also higher in metropolitan areas (8.4 %) compared to rural areas (5.1 %). SAMHSA further reported that the number of US adolescents using cigarettes had dropped from 9.0 to 5.6 % from 2009 to 2013. There were significant drops in usage reported in whites, blacks, and Hispanics.

The detrimental effects of nicotine consumption during pregnancy are well established in the literature. Tobacco use has been demonstrated to cause significant changes within maternal and fetal cell transcriptomes involved in the deregulation of numerous biological processes important for growth and development [3]. It also results in statistically significant reductions of placental vascularization [4]. Both of these findings are related to subsequent fetal morbidities such as small for gestational age infants (SGA), intrauterine growth retardation (IUGR), and low birth weight [5–10]. Smoking includes additional increased risks for the following: cryptorchism in males [11], orofacial clefts [12], asthma and bronchopulmonary hyperreactivity [13, 14], placental abruption [15], fetal malpresentation [16], preterm birth [17, 18] and stillbirth [19, 20].

Demographics and Prevalence

For women abusing tobacco in pregnancy data shows [1]

- One in 5 women smoke prepregnancy
    - Approximately 50 % of women quit smoking by late pregnancy
- Prenatal smokers
    - Higher in <25 years of age; higher among non-Hispanic Whites, American Indians, or Alaska Natives
    - More likely to be low-income and live with a smoker
- Among women who quit during pregnancy, almost ½ relapsed to smoking after delivery

Further barriers to tobacco cessation include a strong culture and a long history of tobacco use. The interplay of values, customs, attitudes, and beliefs all interconnect to work against attempts for tobacco cessation. Each area reinforces the others and any approach to tobacco cessation must account for these interactions (see figure below).

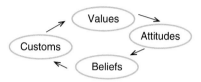

Screening

At prenatal screenings, patients are often asked in their medical history if they use tobacco. However, self-reported tobacco consumption may not be a reliable indicator of total exposure [21]. Studies have shown discrepancy between self-reports of tobacco use and cotinine levels [22, 23]. The issue of the discordance and self-reporting while comparing cotinine levels rests on the frequency of smoking, maternal hydration (with urine testing), renal function, and maternal habitus. The use of maternal saliva to evaluate for cotinine may prove more useful in the future since it is less invasive, less affected by maternal hydration, and more stable as an indicator of level of use.

Another way to measure tobacco usage involves breath analyses of expired carbon monoxide (eCO). These can be less expensive and more rapid than urine drug testing; however, eCO level tests have shown poorer performance at measuring tobacco use than cotinine drugs screens [24]. It has a half-life of 2–8 h, allowing detection of smoking over a 6–24 h period [22]. This reduced half-life would require more frequent testing of eCO (i.e., more trips to the clinic) to obtain more representative measurements of tobacco use. In addition, the process of cigarette smoking is complex. Intake of nicotine during smoking depends on many variables (puff volume, depth of inhalation, the extent of dilution with room air, and the rate and intensity of puffing), all of which can be controlled by the individual [25].

Another alternative involves the major nicotine metabolite, cotinine, which has a half-life of around 16 h, providing a means of assessing tobacco use over a 3 to 4-day period [22]. With a sensitivity of 89.5 % and specificity of 65.3 % [21], cotinine testing can be performed on saliva, urine, or blood samples. A study by Mathai et al. revealed that low birth weights due to smoking have greater correlation with urinary cotinine values than self-reports of tobacco use: "active maternal smoking was associated with a decrease in birth-weight of 12 g for every cigarette smoked in a day while there was a decrease of 25 g in birth-weight for every microgram of cotinine/mg of urinary creatinine" [26]. These values could reveal more information regarding tobacco consumption, which is important to know in the context of pregnancy when studies have noted that there is a direct dose–response association between growth retardation and tobacco exposure [26].

Cessation

Currently, ACOG recommends that every woman who enters prenatal care ought to be asked about tobacco usage and the 5A's utilized [27]:

- *Ask* about tobacco use
- *Advise* to quit (or at least decrease)
- *Assess* willingness to attempt quitting
- *Assist* in quit attempt
- *Arrange* follow-up

As of Oct 2010, the Affordable Care Act mandated that state Medicaid programs (approximately 40 % of births in US) must cover comprehensive tobacco treatment for pregnant women. Promotion of coverage among providers and enrollees is needed to actualize this benefit. One of the foremost strategies has been the use of tobacco quit-line resources. Analysis of quit-line services in ten states during 2006–2008 found:

- 1718 pregnant and 24,321 nonpregnant women enrolled in services.

- Half of pregnant women received self-help materials only.
- Self-reported quit rates at 7 months after enrollment in the subsample were 26.4 % for pregnant women [28].

The military reported similar findings in using a telephone quit-line approach in a cohort of 1298 nonpregnant military patients of both sexes with a 22 % tobacco abstinence rate at 12 months by using a proactive approach with counselors calling the patients to initiate a six-session interview for cessation [29].

A significant number of cofactors/myths surround the implementation of tobacco cessation by women:

- Daily life
- Being pregnant
- Significant others
- Other addictions
- Many thought nicotine was the most dangerous compound in cigarettes.
- Belief that Nicotine Replacement Therapy (NRT) delivered a "pure nicotine" that was worse for the baby than cigarette smoke.

In spite of these barriers, ACOG affirms the following:

- Prenatal care providers deliver a brief counseling session for patients who are willing to try to quit smoking.
- Counseling approaches, such as the 5A's intervention (ask, advise, assess, assist, and arrange), which have been shown to be effective when initiated by healthcare providers.
- Quit lines can be used as support.
- NRT could be considered if behavioral therapy failed; however, cautioned of providing "close supervision" and considering risks of smoking and risks of NRT.

Policy Focus

1. Taxation
2. Youth education and prevention
3. Public/Private partnerships
4. Partnerships in healthcare

Taxation has made significant inroads into the sales of cigarettes in the nation. Studies have shown that as the price of cigarettes rises above $2 a package, the number of cigarettes sold began to decline. Further, as the price exceeded $6 the sales dropped precipitously.

Effective strategies with youth and young adults include:

Cigarettes taxes
100 % smoke-free air laws
Reduce out-of-pocket costs for cessation treatment
Media campaigns

Public and private partnerships have made substantial gains in the establishment of healthier smoke-free environment. Virtually all federal, state, county, and city public buildings are now smoke free. Also, most public malls, stores, and places of business are now smoke free. In the last 15 years, the number of smoke-free restaurants and businesses have increased significantly in the United States. It is estimated that approximately 75 % of all private workplaces are smoke free, with about 30 % of restaurants and approximately 10 % of bars smoke free. Progress continues to be made but further work is necessary.

Most recently, the E-cigarettes present a challenge to present legislation and bans. Since these cigarettes do not produce "smoke" from tobacco and allegedly only water vapor, they are not commonly covered by the present smoking/tobacco bans. The FDA has received reports for possible side effects as well including:

- Pneumonia
- Congestive heart failure
- Disorientation
- Seizure
- Hypotension
- Other health problems

E-cigarettes have undergone no long-term studies and therefore there is no information regarding the potential risks of E-cigarettes when used as intended, how much nicotine or other potentially harmful chemicals are being inhaled during use, or whether there are any benefits associated with using these products. This in particular applies to pregnant patients for which no studies exist regarding the use of E-cigarettes in the context of pregnancy. Nor is there any data on what other chemicals or products might be inhaled with the use of E-cigarettes that cross the placenta to affect the fetus.

Healthcare partners have joined together as well to work with the local providers and politicians to continue to decrease tobacco use as part of healthcare provisions and healthcare benefits.

Pharmacotherapy

Colman et al. 2012 performed a Cochran database evaluation of NRT in the literature. They found six trials of NRT in pregnancy. None of the trials utilized bupropion or varenicline but only evaluated nicotine alone in abstinence/cessation. Coleman et al. 2012 found no difference in cessation in later pregnancy after using NRT as compared to control, RR = 1.33 [0.93–1.91]. They also found no difference in rates of poor birth outcomes (i.e., low birth weight, preterm) between NRT and controls. Significantly, they also found low adherence in NRT in at least one study with only 7 % on therapy at 4 weeks [30].

At present, there is insufficient evidence on efficacy and safety of NRT. Most providers and organizations believe more research is needed to better define the benefit/risk ratio. These concerns are due to the fact that nicotine is a known teratogen. However, it is also known that tobacco includes nicotine plus numerous other chemicals that are injurious to the woman and fetus (cadmium, lead, arsenic, etc).

There is also evidence in the literature whether providers/women would be willing to use NRT during pregnancy. In one study, 30 % of women reported discussing a cessation medication with their obstetric providers [31]. Another study by Tong et al. 2008 found that 3 % of NJ pregnant smokers reported using NRT during pregnancy [32]. ACOG believes that smoking cessation constitutes a vital goal for all pregnant women. So committed to this goal caused ACOG to endorse the web-based course "Smoking Cessation for Pregnancy and Beyond: A Virtual Clinic." The program consists of

1. Web-based training is designed for healthcare professionals to effectively assist pregnant women and women in the childbearing years to quit smoking

   • Physicians, midwives, nurses, health educators, pharmacists, etc...

2. The training program teaches a best practice approach for smoking cessation, the 5A's, and is based on current clinical recommendations from the USPHS and ACOG
3. Program endorsed by ACOG
4. www.smokingcessationandpregnancy.org/

There is significant evidence that encouraging tobacco cessation has real impact in the perinatal outcome in smokers. This impact includes the following:

• Provider efforts have produced quit rates of approximately 10 %.
• Smoking Quit Line has also produced quit rates of 10 %+.
• 5A's quit rates are approximately 20 % for smoking.
• *Quitting* smoking in pregnancy leads to improved birth outcomes, including a 25 % reduction preterm delivery.
• *Cutting down* leads to a 20 % reduction in preterm delivery and a 44 % reduction in NICU admissions.
• Seybold et al. 2012 found that among women in WV, reducing smoking to <8 cigarettes per day had a higher birth weight than those who did not reduce smoking (3.2 vs. 2.9 kg, $p = 0.03$) [33].
• Efforts must be *persistent and consistent* to impact.

Three strategies ought to be employed in every attempt at tobacco cessation within a group or practice:

• Ensure that *patients are urged to quit at every prenatal care visit* and that accurate information on available help is provided. Communicate in a personal way how smoking harms the health of every baby. For patients unable to quit, offer strategies to improve birth outcomes.

- *Launch an education and media campaign* to change language of the term, "low birth weight" and clearly communicate the impact of restricted fetal growth on the developing baby.
- For women who do quit during their pregnancy, provide encouragement *and support for them to remain tobacco-free postpartum.*

References

1. Tong VT, Jones JR, Dietz PM, D'Angelo D, Bombard JM. Trends in smoking before, during, and after pregnancy—Pregnancy Risk Assessment Monitoring System (PRAMS), United States, 31 sites, 2000-2005. MMWR Surveill Summ. 2009;58:1–31.
2. Substance Abuse and Mental Health Services Administration. Behavioral Health Barometer: United States, 2014. HHS Publication No. SMA-15-4895. Rockville: Substance Abuse and Mental Health Services Administration; 2015. p. 4.
3. Votavova H, Dostalova MM, Fejglova K, Vasikova A, Krejcik Z, Pastorkova A, Tabashidze N, Topinka J, Veleminsky Jr M, Sram RJ, Brdicka R. Transcriptome alterations in maternal and fetal cells induced by tobacco smoke. Placenta. 2011;32(10):763–70.
4. Ortigosa S, Friguls B, Joya X, Martinez S, Mariñoso ML, Alameda F, Vall O, Garcia-Algar O. Feto-placental morphological effects of prenatal exposure to drugs of abuse. Reprod Toxicol. 2012;34(1):73–9.
5. Jaddoe VWV, Verburg BO, de Ridder MAJ, Hofman A, Mackenbach JP, Moll HA, Steegers EAP, Witteman JCM, et al. Maternal smoking and fetal growth characteristics in different periods of pregnancy. The generation R study. Am J Epidemiol. 2007;165:1207–15.
6. Ingvarsson RF, Bjarnason AO, Dagbjarsson A, Hardardottir H, Haraldsson A, Thorkelsson T, et al. The effects of smoking in pregnancy on factors influencing fetal growth. Acta Paediatr. 2007;96:383–6.
7. Okah FA, Hoff GL, Dew P, Cai J, et al. Cumulative and residual risks of small for gestational age neonates after changing pregnancy-smoking related behaviors. Am J Perinatol. 2007;24:191–6.
8. Villalbi JR, Salvador J, Cano-Serral G, Rodriguez-Sanz MC, Borrell C. Maternal smoking, social class and outcomes of pregnancy. Paediatr Perinat Epidemiol. 2007;21:441–7.

9. Horta BL, Victora CG, Menezes AM, Halpern R, Barros FC. Low birthweight, preterm births, and intrauterine growth retardation in relation to maternal smoking. Paediatr Perinatal Epidemiol. 1997;11:140–51.

10. Himes SK, Stroud LR, Scheidweiler KB, Niaura RS, Huestis MA. Prenatal tobacco exposure, biomarkers for tobacco in meconium, and neonatal growth outcomes. J Pediatr. 2013;162(5):970–5.

11. Jensen MS, Toft G, Thulstrup AM, Bonde JP, Olsen J, et al. Cryptorchidism according to maternal gestational smoking. Epidemiology. 2007;19(2):220–5.

12. Honein MA, Rasmussen SA, Reefhuis J, Romitti PA, Lammer EJ, Sun L, Correa A, et al. Maternal smoking and environmental tobacco smoke exposure and the risk of orofacial clefts. Epidemiology. 2007;18(2):226–33.

13. Goksor E, Amark M, Alm B, Gustafsson PM, Wennergren G, et al. The impact of pre- and post-natal smoke exposure on future asthma and bronchial hyper-responsiveness. Acta Paediatr. 2007;96:1030–5.

14. Noakes PS, Thomas R, Lane C, Mori TA, Barden AE, Devadason SG, Prescott SL, et al. Association of maternal smoking with increased infant oxidative stress at 3 months of age. Thorax. 2007;62:714–7.

15. Ananth CV, Cnattingius S, et al. Influence of maternal smoking on placental abruption in successive pregnancies: a population-based prospective cohort study in Sweden. Am J Epidemiol. 2007;166:289–95.

16. Talas BB, Altinkaya SO, Talas H, Danisman N, Gungor T. Predictive factors and short-term fetal outcomes of breech presentation: a case-control study. Taiwan J Obstet Gynecol. 2008;47(4):402–7.

17. Andres RL, Day MC. Perinatal complications associated with maternal tobacco use. Semin Neonatal. 2000;5:231–41.

18. Cnattingius S. The epidemiology of smoking during pregnancy; smoking prevalence, maternal characteristics, and pregnancy outcomes. Nicotine Tob Res. 2004;6:125–40.

19. Hogberg L, Cnattingius S, et al. The influence of maternal smoking habits on the risk of subsequent stillbirth: is there a causal relation? BJOG. 2007;114:699–704.

20. Meeker JD, Missmer SA, Vitonis AF, Cramer DW, Hauser R, et al. Risk of spontaneous abortion in women with childhood exposure to parental cigarette smoke. Am J Epidemiol. 2007;166(5):571–5.

21. Britton GR, Brinthaupt J, Stehle JM, James GD. Comparison of self-reported smoking and urinary cotinine levels in a rural preg-

nant population. J Obstet Gynecol Neonatal Nurs. 2004; 33(3):306–11.

22. SRNT Subcommittee on Biochemical Verification. Biochemical verification of tobacco use and cessation. Nicotine Tobacco Res. 2002;4:149–59.

23. Fakhfakh R, Jellouli M, Klouz A, Ben Hamida M, Lakhal M, Belkahia C, Achour N. Smoking during pregnancy and postpartum among Tunisian women. J Matern Fetal Neonatal Med. 2011;24(6):859–62.

24. Kauffman RM, Ferketich AK, Murray DM, Bellair PE, Wewers ME. Measuring tobacco use in a prison population. Nicotine Tob Res. 2010;12(6):582–8.

25. USDHHS. Risks associated with smoking cigarettes with low machine-measured yields of tar and nicotine. Smoking and Tobacco Control Monographs, U.S. Department of Health and Human Services, Public Health Service, National Institutes of Health, National Cancer Institute; 2001.

26. Mathai M, Skinner A, Lawton K, Weindling AM. Maternal smoking, urinary cotinine levels and birth-weight. Aust N Z J Obstet Gynaecol. 1990;30(1):33–6.

27. Committee opinion no. 471: smoking cessation during pregnancy. Obstet Gynecol. 2010;116(5):1241–4.

28. Bombard JM, Farr SL, Dietz PM, Tong VT, Zhang L, Rabius V. Telephone smoking cessation quitline use among pregnant and non-pregnant women. Matern Child Health J. 2013;17(6):989–95.

29. Klesges RC, Ebbert JO, Talcott W, Thomas F, Richey PA, Womack C, Hrysko-Mullen A, Oh J. Efficacy of a tobacco quitline in active duty military and TRICARE beneficiaries: a randomized trial. Mil Med. 2015;180(8):917–25.

30. Coleman T, et al. Pharmacological interventions for promoting smoking cessation during pregnancy. Cochrane Database Syst Rev. 2012;(9):CD010078.

31. Rigotti NA, Prk ER, Chang Y, Regan S. Smoking cessation medication use among pregnant and postpartum smokers. Obstet Gynecol. 2008;111(2):348–55.

32. Tong VT, England LJ, Dietz PM, Asare L. Smoking patterns and use of cessation interventions. Am J Prev Med. 2008;35(4):327–33.

33. Seybold DJ, Broce M, Siegel E, Findley J, Calhoun BC. Smoking in pregnancy in West Virginia: does cessation/reduction improve perinatal outcomes? Matern Child Health J. 2012;16(1):133–8. doi:10.1007/s/10995-010-0730-4.

Chapter 8
Therapeutic Substitution: The West Virginia Success Story

Byron C. Calhoun

Introduction

Substance abuse in pregnancy has well-known deleterious effects on neonates. These effects differ with respect to the substance ingested and can include neonatal abstinence syndrome (NAS), low birth weight, intrauterine fetal demise, and structural abnormalities such as gastroschisis.

The national substance abuse rates have been estimated to be between 2.8 and 19 % [1–3]. These reported rates vary based upon the population screened and the method of screening used. The lowest number reported in the study by Ebrahim and Gfroerer utilized a population survey of the entire United States [1] while the highest rates reported (19 %) by Azadi and Dildy utilized urine toxicology testing [3]. Chasnoff et al. developed a self-reporting screening tool that estimated that 15 % of the population studied continued to use substances of abuse after becoming aware of the pregnancy [2].

Opioid dependence, including methadone maintenance, has been linked to fetal death, growth restriction, preterm

B.C. Calhoun, MD, FACOG, FACS, FASAM, MBA (✉)
Department of Obstetrics and Gynecology, West Virginia
University-Charleston, Charleston, WV, USA
e-mail: Byron.calhoun@camc.org

© Springer International Publishing Switzerland 2016
B.C. Calhoun, T. Lewis (eds.), *Tobacco Cessation and
Substance Abuse Treatment in Women's Healthcare*,
DOI 10.1007/978-3-319-26710-4_8

birth, meconium aspiration, and NAS [4, 5]. NAS may be present in 60–90 % of neonates exposed in utero with up to 70 % of affected neonates with central nervous system irritability that may progress to seizures [5]. Up to 50 % of neonates may experience respiratory issues, feeding problems, and failure to thrive [6]. These issues are present as well in those infants whose mothers' are on methadone maintenance [7]. However, with methadone the onset of NAS may be delayed for several weeks [7]. Some authors recommend 5–8 days of maternal hospitalization while their neonates' undergo observation for NAS [8]. However, most insurance plans will not reimburse for the prolonged uncomplicated maternal stay while awaiting neonatal detoxification.

The incidence of opioid relapse in pregnant opioid abusing women is very high with 41–96 % relapsing. This mirrors the relapse rate of the general population at 1 month of 65–80 % [9, 10]. Over 90 % of patients will relapse at 6 months after medication-assisted withdrawal [11]. Buprenorphine (Subutex™) appears to have no difference in outcomes with regard to treatment of opiate addicted women. The same NAS and neonatal affects are present [12].

Recent work published by Montgomery et al. 2006 compared the performance of meconium samples versus the testing of umbilical cord tissue [13]. This study showed concordance of the testing methods that correlated at or above 90 % for all substances analyzed. Follow-up work included a study in which umbilical cord samples were collected and tested if high-risk criteria for substance abuse were identified. Out of this cohort, 157 of 498 (32 %) cords tested positive for substances of abuse [14]. Stitely et al. 2010 found similar results in their study of cord samples in eight regional hospitals in West Virginia with 146/759 (19.2 %) of umbilical cord samples collected at delivery that were positive for either illicit substances or alcohol [15].

Assessment and Diagnosis of Opioid Dependence

The diagnosis of opioid use disorder is based on criteria outlined in the DSM-5. The criteria describe a problematic pattern of opioid use leading to clinically significant impairment or distress. There are a total of 11 symptoms and severity is specified as either mild (presence of 2–3 symptoms), moderate (presence of 4–5 symptoms), or severe (presence of 6 or more symptoms) within a 12-month period. Opioid use disorder requires that at least two of the 11 criteria be met within a 12-month period: (1) taking opioids in larger amounts or over a longer period of time than intended; (2) having a persistent desire or unsuccessful attempts to reduce or control opioid use; (3) spending excess time obtaining, using, or recovering from opioids; (4) craving for opioids; (5) continuing opioid use causing inability to fulfill work, home, or school responsibilities; (6) continuing opioid use despite having persistent social or interpersonal problems; (7) lack of involvement in social, occupational, or recreational activities; (8) using opioids in physically hazardous situations; (9) continuing opioid use in spite of awareness of persistent physical or psychological problems; (10) tolerance, including need for increased amounts of opioids or diminished effect with continued use at the same amount—as long as the patient is not taking opioids under medical supervision; and (11) withdrawal manifested by characteristic opioid withdrawal syndrome or taking opioids to relieve or avoid withdrawal symptoms—while not taking opioids under medical supervision [16].

Immediate clinical priority ought to include identifying and making appropriate referral for any urgent or emergent medical or psychiatric problem(s), including drug related impairment or overdose. The medical history should include screening for concomitant medical conditions, infectious diseases (hepatitis, HIV, and tuberculosis [TB]), acute trauma, and pregnancy. Physical examination should be completed as a comprehensive portion of the thorough assessment process. The prescriber (the clinician authorizing the use of a medication for the treatment of opioid use disorder) ought to conduct this physical examination him/herself, or, in accordance with the ASAM Standards, ensure that a recent and accurate physical examination is found within the patient medical record prior to the initiation of a new medication for the treatment of his/her addiction.

Initial laboratory testing consists of a complete blood count, liver function tests, hepatitis C and HIV. Expanded panels of testing for TB and sexually transmitted infections should also be considered. Hepatitis A & B vaccination should be offered, if appropriate.

The assessment of women presents special considerations regarding their reproductive health. All women of reproductive age should be tested for pregnancy, and all women of childbearing potential and age should be counseled regarding methods of contraception, since increase in fertility may result from effective opioid use disorder treatment.

Patients being evaluated for addiction involving opioid use, and/or for possible medication use in the treatment of opioid use disorder, should undergo (or have completed) an assessment of mental health status and possible psychiatric disorders (as outlined in the ASAM Standards).

Opioid use often co-exists with other substance related disorders. An inquiry into past and current substance use and an evaluation of all of the substances involved in the addiction should be conducted.

The use of marijuana, stimulants, or other addictive substances should deter opioid use disorder treatment. However, evidence demonstrates patients who actively abuse other non-prescribed substances during opioid use disorder treatment have a poorer prognosis. The co-abuse of benzodiazepines and other sedative hypnotics may be a reason to suspend agonist treatment due to safety concerns related to respiratory depression and death.

A tobacco questionnaire and counseling on tobacco cessation ought to be completed routinely for all patients, including those who present for evaluation and treatment of opioid use disorder.

ASAM Standards also suggest an assessment of social and environmental factors be conducted to identify facilitators and barriers to addiction treatment, and especially for pharmacotherapy. Prior to a decision to initiate a course of pharmacotherapy for the patient with opioid use disorder, the patient should receive a multidimensional assessment in fidelity with The ASAM Criteria: Treatment Criteria for Addictive, Substance-Related, and Co-occurring Conditions (the "ASAM Criteria"). Addiction may be considered a bio-psycho-social-spiritual illness, for which the use of medication(s) is but only one component of overall treatment.

Diagnosis of opioid use disorder is confirmed by the provider prescribing medications, and who recommends medication use. Diagnosis must be obtained before pharmacotherapy for opioid use disorder commences. Opioid use disorder is primarily diagnosed on the history given by the patient and a thorough assessment including a physical examination. Validated clinical scales that measure withdrawal symptoms, for example, the Objective Opioid Withdrawal Scale (OOWS), the Subjective Opioid Withdrawal Scale (SOWS), and the Clinical Opioid Withdrawal Scale (COWS), may be used to assist in the evaluation of patients with opioid use disorder. Urine drug testing during assessment process, and frequently during treatment, is recommended. The frequency of drug testing is determined by multiple factors: patient compliance, the type of treatment including medications, and the treatment setting: inpatient or outpatient.

Pregnant women constitute a special population in opioid use disorders. In the evaluation of pregnant women for opioid use disorder, obstetrical conditions that require immediate referral for clinical evaluation should be determined. This may include referral to a maternal–fetal medicine specialist. Complete medical examination and psychosocial assessment is paramount when evaluating pregnant women for opioid use disorder. Obstetricians and gynecologists should be alert to signs and symptoms of opioid use disorder [17]. Pregnant women with opioid use disorder often seek prenatal care late in pregnancy, miss appointments, experience poor weight gain, may have small for gestational age fetuses, undergo preterm labor/delivery, have placental abruption, or exhibit signs of withdrawal or intoxication.

Psychosocial treatment should be offered in the treatment of pregnant women with opioid use disorder. Counseling and testing for HIV should be a routine part of care. Testing for hepatitis B and C along with liver function is highly encouraged. Hepatitis A and B vaccination should be considered for those whose hepatitis serology is negative. Urine drug testing may be utilized to detect or confirm suspected opioid and other drug use with informed consent from the mother, realizing that there may be adverse legal and social consequences of her use. State laws differ on reporting substance use during pregnancy. Laws that penalize women for use and for obtaining treatment may prevent women from obtaining prenatal care and worsen outcomes. A comprehensive assessment of mental health, including determination of the patient's present mental health status, should evaluate whether the patient is emotionally and psychologically stable enough for opioid therapy. Patients with suicidal or homicidal ideation ought to be referred immediately for treatment and hospitalization. Management of patients at risk for suicide should include: decreasing imminent risks; modulating underlying factors associated with suicidal ideation; ongoing monitoring of psychological status, and follow-up by mental health professionals. As in a non-addicted population, patients with psychiatric disorders should be asked about suicidal ideation, suicidal plans/intent, and behavior. Patients with a history of suicidal ideation or suicide attempts should have opioid use disorder, and psychiatric medication use, monitored closely by the healthcare team. Frequent visits may be necessary to insure compliance and good clinical outcomes. Evaluation for psychiatric disorder should occur at the very beginning of agonist or antagonist treatment prior to initiating drug therapy. Reassessment using a detailed mental status examination should occur after stabilization with methadone, buprenorphine, or naltrexone. Pharmacotherapy in conjunction with psychosocial treatment should be considered for patients with opioid use disorder and a co-existing psychiatric disorder. Providers caring for women should be acutely aware of potential interaction between medications used to treat co-occurring psychiatric conditions and opioid use disorder. Possible community treatment should be considered for patients with co-occurring schizophrenia and opioid use disorder who have a recent history of, or are at risk of, repeated hospitalization or homelessness.

Adolescents and Opioid Use Disorders

The American Academy of Pediatrics categorizes adolescence as the totality of three developmental stages—puberty to adulthood—which occur between 11 and 21 years of age. Eleven young people within this age group—adolescents—present for treatment with a broad spectrum of opioid use disorder severity and with co-occurring medical and psychiatric illness. Therefore, providers will need to respond with a full range of treatment options, including pharmacotherapy. This is especially challenging in the pregnant adolescent. Unfortunately, there is limited evidence regarding the efficacy of opioid withdrawal management in adolescents [18]. Pharmacological therapies have been almost exclusively developed through research with adult populations and not adolescents [19]. The treatment of adolescents with opioid use disorder presents many unique medical, legal, and ethical dilemmas that may complicate treatment. Due to these unique issues, adolescents with opioid use disorder often benefit from services designed specifically for them. Also, the family, provided they are not part of the problem, should be involved in treatment whenever possible. The "Confidentiality in Treatment" is one issue that may be of particular importance to consider in the treatment of adolescents. Adolescents themselves have reported that they are less likely to seek substance use disorder treatment if services are not confidential [20]. Confidential care, particularly with respect to sensitive issues such as reproductive health and substance use, has become a well-established practice [21, 22]. These issues are an area governed by both Federal and state laws. Moreover, defined age ranges of "adolescence" vary. A variety of clinical and legal responsibilities may be involved if confronted by a young person's request for confidentiality. More than half of the states in the United States, by law, permit adolescents less than 18 years of age to consent to substance use disorder treatment without parental consent. State law should also be consulted. An additional resource in decision-making regarding the implications on coordination of care, effectiveness of treatment without parental communication, and other key issues are more completely elucidated in a publication of the Substance Abuse and Mental Health Services Administrations (SAMHSA), Center for Substance Abuse Treatment, Treatment Improvement Protocol (TIP) #33 [23].

Pharmacotherapeutic options for adolescents include the opioid agonists (methadone and buprenorphine) and antagonists (naltrexone) for treatment of opioid use disorder in adolescents. However, efficacy studies for these medications have largely been conducted in adults. Their recommended use is based on the consensus opinion of the Guideline Committee [24]. There are virtually no data comparing the relative effectiveness of these treatments in adolescents with adults. Methadone and buprenorphine are the agonist medications indicated for the treatment of patients who are aged 18 years and older. The Federal code on opioid treatment—42 CFR § 8.12—offers an exception for patients aged 16 and 17, who have a documented history of at least two prior unsuccessful withdrawal management attempts, and have parental consent [25].

There are no controlled trials evaluating the efficacy of agonists and partial agonists in adolescents, such as methadone for the treatment of opioid use disorder in adolescents under the age of 18. Descriptive trials support the apparent effectiveness of treatment with methadone in supporting treatment retention in adolescent heroin users [26]. The usefulness of treatment with buprenorphine with heroin use in adolescents has been demonstrated in two RCTs. Studies have, however, not included adolescents under the age of 16 [27,28]. Buprenorphine is not US FDA-approved for use in patients less than 16 years old. Buprenorphine is more likely to be available in programs targeting older adolescents and young adults. No direct comparison of the efficacy buprenorphine versus methadone has been conducted in adolescent populations.

The opioid antagonist naltrexone may be considered for young adults aged 18 years and older who have opioid use disorder. Naltrexone has no physical dependence and is simpler to discontinue usage. Oral naltrexone may be particularly useful for adolescents who report a shorter duration of opioid use. Extended-release injectable naltrexone is administered monthly and may be delivered on an outpatient basis. Only one small case series demonstrated the efficacy of extended-release injectable naltrexone in adolescents [29]. The safety, efficacy, and pharmacokinetics of extended-release injectable naltrexone have not been established in the adolescent population to allow its use without close observation.

Psychosocial treatment is recommended in the treatment of all adolescents with opioid use disorder. Useful treatments based on the consensus opinion of the Guideline Committee include family intervention approaches, vocational support, and behavioral interventions to incrementally reduce use. Holistic risk-reduction interventions emphasizing healthy life-choices, which promote practices to reduce infection, are particularly important in the prevention of sexually transmitted infections and blood-borne viruses. Treatment of concomitant psychiatric conditions is also critically necessary in this population. Adolescents often benefit from specialized treatment facilities that provide multiple services combined in a single, focal setting.

Pregnancy and Opioid Use Disorder

Care for pregnant women with opioid use disorder should be considered a particularly vulnerable population and ideally be comanaged by an obstetrician and an addiction specialist physician. Unfortunately, in many areas, this is simply not possible due to a paucity of trained addictions specialists and active programs for pregnant patients. As per normal procedures, release of information forms needs to be completed to ensure communication among healthcare providers.

The common dictum is that pregnant women who are physically dependent on opioids should receive treatment using methadone or buprenorphine monoproduct rather than withdrawal management or abstinence. However, substitution, without working toward abstinence from opioids, does not address the problems of NAS in the neonates after delivery. As previously noted, methadone and buprenorphine both have significant issues with NAS.

If treatment with methadone is initiated, it should commence as early as possible during pregnancy. Hospitalization during initiation of methadone and treatment with buprenorphine may be advisable due to the potential for adverse events, especially in the third trimester. Generally, adverse events may be avoided by routine employment of fetal monitoring protocols with non-stress testing or biophysical profiles to ensure fetal well-being. If an inpatient setting is chosen, methadone should be started at a dose range of 20–30 mg/day. Incremental doses of 5–10 mg may be given every 3–6 h, as needed, to treat withdrawal symptoms. After clinical induction, clinicians may increase the methadone dose in 5–10-mg increments per week if needed. The goal is to maintain the lowest dose that controls withdrawal symptoms and decreases the desire to use additional opioids. Twice daily dosing appears more effective and has fewer side effects than single daily dosing. However, it may not be practical if the methadone is dispensed in an outpatient clinic.

Obstetrician/Gynecologists caring for opioid use disorder pregnant patients should be aware that the pharmacokinetics of methadone clearance is affected by pregnancy. With advancing gestational age, plasma levels of methadone progressively decrease and clearance increases. Increased or split doses may be needed as pregnancy progresses. After child birth, doses may need to be adjusted back to lower levels.

Buprenorphine monoproduct has become a possible alternative to methadone for pregnant women. There appear to be no concerns with the combination buprenorphine/naloxone formulation but there is inadequate data to recommend its use at this time. If a woman becomes pregnant while she is receiving naltrexone, it appears reasonable to stop the medication if the patient and doctor agree that the risk of relapse is low. If the patient is highly concerned about relapse and wishes to continue naltrexone, she should be informed about the risks of staying on naltrexone. Informed consent for ongoing treatment should be obtained with a signed document of understanding. If the patient wishes to discontinue naltrexone, but then reports relapse to opioid use, it may be reasonable to consider treatment with methadone or treatment with buprenorphine. Naloxone therapy is generally not recommended for use in pregnant women with opioid use disorder except in life-threatening overdose. Mothers receiving methadone and buprenorphine monoproduct for the treatment of opioid use disorders may breastfeed without any concerns to the neonate since only small amounts of drug are released in breast milk.

West Virginia

The number of newborns treated for NAS has increased dramatically in West Virginia. In data collected from the Cabell Huntington Hospital in Huntington, WV, the number of neonates treated for NAS increased from 25 in 2003 to 70 in 2007 [30]. The cost difference in the care of an otherwise healthy neonate with NAS compared to a normal full-term healthy neonate was estimated to be $3934 in the Cabell-Huntington cohort. Because of the added costs associated with the increased risk of prematurity, the average cost of all infants with NAS was $36,000 compared to $2000 for a normal neonate [30].

Staff of Charleston Area Medical Center (CAMC), West Virginia's only free-standing Women and Children's Hospital, knew they were providing care to around 130 babies born annually with positive substance screens (4 % deliveries) based on risk factor screening at the time of presentation and delivery. However, the actual numbers were much more startling. We obtained new information for our hospital from Stitely et al. 2010 that indicated a much higher abuse rate [15]. A cross-sectional hospital study was initiated in eight West Virginia hospitals in 2009 to examine the prevalence of substance use in pregnant patients at delivery and CAMC participated [15]. Segments of umbilical cords were collected anonymously from 759 deliveries (regardless of risk factors) at the eight regional hospitals during the month of August, 2009. A reference laboratory screened all cord segments for the presence of substances using commercially available enzyme-linked immunoabsorbent (ELISA) kits, with confirmatory testing by gas chromatography/mass spectrometry were used for 6 of the drugs. Buprenorphine was tested using liquid chromatography/mass spectrometry (LCMSMS). Phosphatidylethanol (a metabolite of ethanol testing was based on high-pressure liquid chromatography/mass spectrometry (HPLCMS). CAMC's overall positive screening rate was 16 % for non-prescribed and illicit drugs and 8 % for alcohol) out of the total of 133 patients screened. These findings of positive screening by cord blood samples were four times higher than our rate of 4 % when we screened based on risk factors. In addition, results from the study indicated that multiple drug use was common [15].

Most recent data from CAMC presented by Hensel et al. 2012, found with universal urine screening for illicit substances in the CAMC obstetric and gynecologic residency clinic in West Virginia, that, 32 % of pregnant patients at CAMC were positive for illicit substances including 11 % positive for multiple substances [31].

Prior to the August, 2009 study, CAMC received a grant in the spring of 2009 from the Appalachian Regional Commission to address the alleged 4 % substance abuse rate by risk factor screening alone for delivery at our institution and explore the issues in substance abuse in pregnancy as part of their initiative for "Partnering for a Drug-Free America." The proceeds from the grant were utilized by the Drug Addicted Mom and Babies (DAMB) task force which had been developed 2 years prior, to address the growing issue of women and babies affected by addiction and substance abuse during pregnancy and the time of delivery.

The DAMB task force is a multidisciplinary group including nursing personnel from the inpatient obstetrical and NICU areas and the outpatient clinical areas, a substance abuse counselor, physicians, a nursing educator, and a research associate. The director of a local halfway house for women recovering from substance abuse is also included on the task force for community representation.

Outpatient Therapeutic Substitution

In response to the substance abuse issue among pregnant women, an outpatient treatment program with therapeutic substitution was created to provide individual and group based substance abuse intervention with a certified substance abuse counselor (see Appendix 1 for dosing). Patients were identified for substance abuse by referral, previous substance abuse history, and urine drug screening.

The substance abuse literature suggested the avoidance of detoxification during the second and third trimesters of pregnancy due to concerns about harms to the fetus [4, 32]. Recent literature, however, does not substantiate these claims [5, 32–35]. Luty et al. 2003 studied 101 opiate-dependent women who underwent a 21-day gradual opiate withdrawal with no adverse effects found [35]. Stewart et al. 2013 utilized a slow methadone inpatient taper for pregnant inpatients [36]. They found that in 53/96 (56 %) of patients could successfully be detoxified. Further, the hospital stays for those with inpatient detoxification lasted 10 days longer than those who did not detoxify (25 versus 15 days). They also found that maternal demographics and drug histories did not influence successful inpatient detoxification. Their findings suggested that opiate detoxification ought to be offered to all pregnant women willing to undergo detoxification [36].

Finally, Hensel et al. 2015 cared for 92 screen-positive patients and achieved abstinence in 39/92 (42 %) patients at delivery with outpatient management with oral therapeutic opioid substitution with decreasing dosages while including contingency addictions care by a certified addictions specialist. [37] They found collaborative and intense group therapy with a certified addictions counselor was a mainstay of successful achievement of abstinence [38].

Patients in the CAMC resident clinics who received obstetrical care from 6/30/2010–3/31/2013 were enrolled in our multidisciplinary care in the CAMC obstetrics and gynecology resident outpatient obstetric clinic areas. Our plan of care included a certified substance abuse counselor, obstetrical staff/resident physicians, trained nursing personnel, and a nursing educator. Key in the management of our obstetrical patients' care was routine screening of patients' initial urine for illicit and non-prescribed substances. All patients who tested positive for non-prescribed, or illicit substances, were enrolled in our abstinence-based addictions program including our contingency management program for substance abuse staffed by a certified addictions specialist. The CAMC program consisted of a 12-week course of group therapy and addictions counseling by our certified addictions counselor. Weekly visits to the high-risk obstetrical clinic were included. Testing of patients' urine for illicit substances continued throughout their obstetrical care. Patients who took opiates, and were at risk for acute opiate withdrawal, received therapeutic substitution with oral opioid medications to obtain abstinence. The program used medical care including outpatient therapeutic substitution with decreasing dosages of opiates with weekly group meetings, which focused on improving coping skills and increasing distress tolerance. Patient's urines were tested weekly to insure compliance with care and dosage verification by mass spectrometry analysis with patient BMI and urine specific gravity.

The therapy component of the program consists of both psycho-educational and cognitive-behavioral therapy. Information is provided on the disease concept of addiction, Step One, the recovery process, relapse prevention, and the effects of drugs on the baby. A contingency management program, an evidence-based practice with roots in Motivational Interviewing, was utilized to keep patients engaged in their abstinence process. Contingency management therapies are a type of psychosocial intervention where the clients receive rewards in the form of vouchers or prizes if they demonstrate changed behaviors. Data supports contingency management therapy in cocaine and opioid abuse [39, 40]. It has also been shown to be effective in the vulnerable populations of co-occurring psychological disorders and in pregnant women.

Analysis of the delivery outcomes in patients screening positive for substance abuse in pregnancy was performed for our CAMC patients. Variables analyzed from urine drug data were linked to addiction intervention program.

Results of Outpatient Therapeutic Substitution in West Virginia

Inclusion criteria were met by 1164 patients in our CAMC tertiary medical center women's health clinic. Tobacco use is around 50 % and alcohol around 7 % in the clinic. Three hundred fifteen (27 %) women tested positive on urine drug screens for substances. Three hundred nineteen (27 %) women tested positive on urine drug screens for substances. Substances found in decreasing frequency: marijuana—241 (76 %), opiates—68 (21 %), benzodiazepines—32 (10 %), methadone—17 (5 %), cocaine—15 (5 %), and amphetamines—10 (3 %). Forty-three (13 %) women tested positive for more than one substance. Of the 68 women positive for prenatal opiate use, 51 gave birth at our facility of which 21 (41 %) achieved abstinence. As a result of abstinence at birth, there was an estimated savings of over $700,000 in abstinence therapy ($34,000 per neonate) in NICU costs alone.

Postoperative and Postpartum Care in Opioid Patients

A final word must be shared in the care of opioid tolerant pregnant patients that often goes unnoticed: postoperative and postpartum care. The care of opioid tolerant patients must consider:

- Pain is frequently undertreated
- May require longer postoperative treatment
- Usually require more than replacement dose
- Ought to avoid antagonist/agonist or partial agonist meds (buprenorphine, butorphanol, pentazocine)

Generally should continue previous meds or equivalent chronic pain medications in the acute postoperative stages. Usually increase postoperative, procedural dose, etc. by 25–50 % of baseline dosing. Key questions to ask the opioid tolerant/addicted patients are what medications they are receiving (dose, duration, route) and whether or not they are taking any neuropathic meds (neurontin, etc).

For postoperative pain in opioid tolerant individuals, the following is suggested to insure adequate pain coverage:

1. Calculate daily preoperative oral dose then convert to IV morphine equivalents
2. Give 50 % of calculated daily morphine equivalent as background infusion
3. Adjust per PCA pump protocols

For acute pain relief in postoperative pain in opioid addict in recovery (not taking any opioids), consider pain relief as below:

- Utilize local or regional blocks when able
- Don't force meds on patients

- If possible, avoid drug of abuse
- In emergencies, use what you need
- Optimize nonsteroidals (i.e., toradol IM/IV)
- Start with standard opiate doses

Further considerations for opioid tolerant-opioid maintenance therapy patients (on opioid medications) must be dealt
with for postoperative pain. Methadone patients should be
treated:

- Treated the same as chronic opioid patients.
- Maintain their baseline of methadone and supplement
  with standard opioid dose and titrate accordingly. May
  give IM methadone as well.
- If unable to tolerate PO/IM, convert to IV morphine
  equivalents. Give 25–50 % of total dose as baseline.
- Adjust according to PCA protocols.
- Avoid partial agonists or opioid antagonists.

Buprenorphine (Suboxone/Subutex) ought to be prescribed to maintain postoperative pain relief by considering
these principles:

- $\times 30$–$\times 40$ more potent than morphine on an mg per mg
  basis
- Generally less hemodynamic effects than traditional
  opiates
- May dose SQ
- Dose every 6–8 h

Dosing for buprenorphine for postoperative pain relief
should include:

- Dosing for pain 3–4 times per day SC/IV.
- Patient may use own SL medication (if approved by treat-
  ment doctor) administrated by nurse.
- Good for same day surgery patients as well as hospitalized.
- Dose 0.3 mg SC/IV every 6–8 h for postoperative pain.
- Can use standard scheduled dose of IV morphine/hydro-
  morphine Q4–6 h and adjust as needed.

The pain relief doses for buprenorphine may be converted to morphine dose equivalents by using the following information:

- Total mg of buprenorphine $SL \times 50$ = total daily oral morphine dose.
- 8 mg/2 mg/day (1 strip) $\times 50$ = 400 mg/day oral morphine.
- Initiate 25–50 % of calculated dose as a PCA baseline, then adjust per protocol.
- 100–200 mg/day divided Q4–6 h+ prn doses oral morphine.

To assist in the postoperative care of our opioid tolerant and opioid naïve patients, we developed order sets for labor and delivery for intrapartum pain relief, post-vaginal delivery pain relief, and postoperative (cesarean section) pain relief (see Appendices 2–4). These order sets are provided for illustrative purposes to allow a framework for development of order sets pertinent to the healthcare system and pertinent to the local practices of the various providers.

References

1. Ebrahim SH, Gfroerer J. Pregnancy-related substance use in the United States during 1996-1998. Obstet Gynecol. 2003;101(2): 374–9.
2. Chasnoff IJ, McGourty RF, Bailey GW, Hutchins E, Lightfoot SO, Pawson LL, Fahey C, May B, Brodie P, McCulley L, Campbell J. The 4P's Plus screen for substance use in pregnancy: clinical application and outcomes. J Perinatol. 2005;25(6):368–74.
3. Azadi A, Dildy III GA. Universal screening for substance abuse at the time of parturition. Am J Obstet Gynecol. 2008;198(5):e30–2. Epub 2008 Feb 14.
4. Rementeria JL, Nunag NN. Narcotic withdrawal in pregnancy. Am J Obstet Gynecol. 1973;116:1152–6.
5. Hoegerman G, Schnoll SH. Methadone maintenance and withdrawal in pregnant opioid addicts. Clin Perinatol. 1991;18:51–76.
6. Briggs GG, Freeman RK, Yaffee SJ. Drugs in pregnancy and lactation. Baltimore: Williams and Wilkins; 1994. p. 557–8.

7. Cooper JR, Altman F, Brown BS, Czechowicz D, editors. Research on the treatment of narcotic addiction: State of the art. (NIDA Research Monograph 83-1201). Rockville: US Department of Health and Human Services; 1983.

8. Andres RL, Jones KL. Social and illicit drug use in pregnancy. In: Creasy RK, Resnick R, editors. Maternal-fetal medicine. Philadelphia: Saunders; 1994. p. 191–2.

9. Winklbaur B, Kopf N, Ebner N, Jung E, Thau K, Fischer G. Treating pregnant women dependent on opioids is not the same as treating pregnancy and opioid dependence: a knowledge synthesis for better treatment for women and neonates. Addiction. 2008;103:1429–40.

10. Chutuape MA, Jasinski DR, Fingerhood MI, Stitzer ML. One, three, and six month outcomes following brief inpatient opioid detoxification. Am J Drug Alcohol Abuse. 2001;27:19–44.

11. Gossop M, Green L, Phillips G, Bradley B. Lapse, relapse, and survival among opiate addicts immediately after treatment: a prospective follow-up study. Br J Psychiatry. 1989;154:348–53.

12. Jones HE, Johnson RE, Jasinski DR, O'Grady KE, Chisholm CA, Choo RE, Crocetti M, Dudas R, Harrow C, Huestis MA, Jansson LM, Lantz M, Lester BM, Milio L. Buprenorphine versus methadone in the treatment of pregnant opioid-dependent patients: effects on the neonatal abstinence syndrome. Drug Alcohol Depend. 2004;79:1–10.

13. Montgomery D, Plate C, Alder SC, Jones M, Jones J, Christensen RD. Testing for fetal exposure to illicit drugs using umbilical cord tissue vs meconium. J Perinatol. 2006;26(1):11–4.

14. Montgomery DP, Plate CA, Jones M, Jones J, Rios R, Lambert DK, Schumtz N, Wiedmeier SE, Burnett J, Ail S, Brandel D, Maichuck G, Durham CA, Henry E, Christensen RD. Using umbilical cord tissue to detect fetal exposure to illicit drugs: a multicentered study in Utah and New Jersey. J Perinatol. 2008;28(11):750–3. Epub 2008 Jul 3.

15. Stitely ML, Calhoun BC, Maxwell S, Nerhood R, Chaffin D. Prevalence of drug use in pregnant West Virginia patients. W V Med J. 2010;105:48–52.

16. American Psychiatric Association: diagnostic and statistical manual of mental disorders. 5th edition. Arlington: American Psychiatric Association; 2013.

17. American College of Obstetricians Committee Opinion Number 524: Opioid abuse, dependence, and addiction ion pregnancy; May 2012 (reaffirmed 2014).

18. Minozzi S, Amato L, Bellisario C, et al. Detoxification treatments for opiate dependent adolescents. Cochrane Database Syst Rev. 2014;(4):CD006749.
19. Minozzi S, Amato L, Bellisario C, et al. Maintenance treatments for opiate-dependent adolescents. Cochrane Database Syst Rev. 2014;(6):CD007210.
20. Ford CA, Millstein SG, Halpern-Felsher BL, et al. Influence of physician confidentiality assurances on adolescents' willingness to disclose information and seek future health care. A randomized controlled trial. J Am Med Assoc. 1997;278:1029–34.
21. Hallfors DD, Waller MW, Ford CA, et al. Adolescent depression and suicide risk: association with sex and drug behavior. Am J Prev Med. 2004;27:224–31.
22. Weddle M, Kokotailo PK. Confidentiality and consent in adolescent substance abuse: an update. Virtual Mentor. 2005;7(3).
23. Substance Abuse and Mental Health Services Administration. Treatment improvement protocol series 33: treatment for stimulant use disorders. Rockville: Substance Abuse and Mental Health Services Administration; 1999.
24. American Society of Addiction Medicine: The ASAM National Practice guideline for the use of medications in the treatment of addiction involving opioid use; June 2015.
25. Substance Abuse and Mental Health Services Administration. Federal guidelines for opioid treatment, 2013 revision, draft. Available at: http://www.dpt.samhsa.gov/pdf/FederalGuidelinesforOpioidTreatment5-62013revisiondraft_508.pdf.
26. Hopfer CJ, Khuri E, Crowley TJ, et al. Adolescent heroin use: a review of the descriptive and treatment literature. J Subst Abuse Treat. 2002;23:231–7.
27. Substance Abuse and Mental Health Services Administration. Treatment improvement protocol series 45: detoxification and substance abuse treatment. Rockville: Substance Abuse and Mental Health Services Administration; 2006.
28. Woody GE, Poole SA, Subramaniam G, et al. Extended vs short-term buprenorphine-naloxone for treatment of opioid-addicted youth: a randomized trial. J Am Med Assoc. 2008;300:2003–11.
29. Fishman MJ, Winstanley EL, Curran E, et al. Treatment of opioid dependence in adolescents and young adults with extended release naltrexone: preliminary case-series and feasibility. Addiction. 2010;105:1669–76.
30. Baxter FR, Nerhood R, Chaffin D. Characterization of babies discharged from Cabell Huntington Hospital during the calen-

dar year 2005 with the diagnoses of neonatal abstinence syndrome. W V Med J. 2009;105(2):16–21.

31. Hensel S, Seybold D, Lewis T, Burgess D, Casto A, Calhoun BC. Substance Abuse in Pregnancy: Role of Universal Urine Drug Screening and Addiction Therapy in West Virginia. Poster presented in 16th World Congress on Controversies in Obstetrics, Gynecology, and Infertility (COGI), Singapore, 19–22 July 2012.

32. Finnegan JP. Treatment issues for opioid dependent women during the perinatal period. J Psychoactive Drugs. 1991;23:191–202.

33. Jarvis MAE, Schnoll SH. Methadone maintenance and withdrawal in pregnant opioid addicts. In: Chiang CN, Finnegan LP, editors. Medication development for the treatment of pregnant addicts and their infants (NIDA Monograph 149). Washington, DC: US Department of Health and Human Services; 1995. p. 58–77.

34. Dashe JS, Jackson GL, Olscher DA, Zane EH, Wendel GD. Opioid detoxification in pregnancy. Obstet Gynecol. 1998;92:854–8.

35. Luty J, Nikolaou V, Bearn J. Is opiate detoxification unsafe in pregnancy? J Subst Abuse Treat. 2003;24:363–7.

36. Stewart RD, Nelson DB, Adhikari EH, McIntire DD, Roberts SW, Dashe JS, Sheffield JS. The obstetrical and neonatal impact of maternal opioid detoxification in pregnancy. Am J Obstet Gynecol. 2013;209:267.e1–5.

37. Hensel S, Seybold D, Lewis T, Burgess D, Casto A, Barnes A, Calhoun BC. Substance Abuse in Pregnancy: role of Universal Urine Drug Screening and Outpatient Addiction Therapy in West Virginia. Poster Presented in 62nd Annual Meeting of Society for Reproductive Investigation (SGR), San Francisco, 26–28 March 2015.

38. Silsby H, Tennat FS. Short-term, ambulatory detoxification of opiate addicts using methadone. Int J Addict. 1974;9:167–70.

39. Petry NM, Alessi SM, Marx J, Austin M, Tardif M. Vouchers versus prizes: contingency management treatment of substance use disorders: a meta-analysis. J Consult Clin Psychol. 2005;73:1005–14.

40. Petry NM, Alessi SM, Hanson T, Sierra S. Randomized trial of contingent prizes versus vouchers in cocaine-using methadone patients. J Consult Clin Psychol. 2007;75:983–91.

Index

© Springer International Publishing Switzerland 2016   157
B.C. Calhoun, T. Lewis (eds.), *Tobacco Cessation and
Substance Abuse Treatment in Women's Healthcare*,
DOI 10.1007/978-3-319-26710-4